HOW
MEN
HAVE
babies

HOW
MEN
HAVE
babies

THE PREGNANT FATHER'S
SURVIVAL GUIDE

ALANTHICKE

JODERE
GROUP
San Diego, California

JODERE
GROUP

P.O. Box 910147
San Diego, California 92191-0147
800.569.1002
w w w . j o d e r e . c o m

CIP data available from the Library of Congress

ISBN 1-58872-060-8
06 05 04 03   4 3 2 1
First printing, May 2003

PRINTED IN CANADA

EDITORIAL SUPERVISION BY CHAD EDWARDS

BOOK DESIGN BY CHARLES MCSTRAVICK

CONTENTS

INTRODUCTION

First of all, I want to thank you for buying this book. I am now that much closer to a best seller and my kid's college fund appreciates the contribution. This is a book about pregnancy from a man's perspective, intended to get him involved early and fully.

By way of introduction, let me say that the chances are I am not like you. I am not married. If you ever hear that I have written a book about marriage, put it down, walk away slowly, and nobody will get hurt.

I have married twice and been a Dad three times, which makes me "plus one" in hockey terms. My first time has to be deemed a success—you should be allowed one Marriage Mulligan in Hollywood—with a 13-year run and two glorious children.

My second marriage, in retrospect, probably happened because we both wanted a baby and we crossed our fingers that the other "marriage stuff" would fall into place. It didn't.

But you can't blame a guy for trying. And the pregnancy period was as full and rich as two people could hope for. The baby boy was reason enough for getting married, and single parenting has worked out for all three of us, if not the recommended first choice.

Some of the humor in this book may explain why two women are no longer with me. All I remember is we had a lot of laughs—you can ask their lawyers—and my stories are meant to help you break the ice if humor is one of the victims of your first, nervous pregnancy. Hopefully, you'll see that we're all the same when it comes to this job and the fear and excitement that come with it. I will, therefore, refer often to the women with whom I shared memories that will never fade for any of us. As it should be.

So, please forgive that imperfection on my résumé—marriage to me is like the Justice System . . . I believe in it, I just don't understand it sometimes—and trust that I know whereof I speak on the father front. I have read many books on the subject. I have consulted experts and done my research and most importantly, I have been there, done that. I have loved and suffered and been *ecstasized* by my kids and have formulated my thesis accordingly.

I have tried to make this read chock-full of information and fun. I hope it works for you.

DISCLAIMER

- **More than 10,000 babies are born every day in the United States.**

- **The average couple is married for three years before their first pregnancy.**

- **The average age of the parents is 28.4 years. (He's 31; she's 27.)**

You've read about couplehood and babyhood. But the one neighborhood left uncovered is the one that starts the ball rolling: *pregnanthood.*

How Men Have Babies aims to be the pregnant father's guide book. The narrative is presented chronologically, following your baby's momentum as he carries you from month to month.

Expect an occasional episode of sampling, the current musical term for plagiarism, the art of stealing material: I prefer to call it *Internet Awareness*, and I promise nothing is stolen intentionally from any singular author whose identity we could trace.

In addition, I have solicited anecdotes from some well-known personalities whose voices will provide a welcome relief from my own.

They include:

- **TOM ARNOLD, actor**

- **DAVE BARRY, hilarious dad**

- **CORBIN BERNSEN, actor and president of Famous Fathers, Inc. (self-proclaimed)**

- **BARRY GIBB, legendary Bee Gee**

- **KATHIE LEE GIFFORD, songbird**

- **CUBA GOODING, JR., Oscar winner**

- **WAYNE GRETZKY, puck god**

- **JERRY HALL, model and senior rocker's ex**

- **JOANNA KERNS, *Growing Pains* wife and international sex symbol**

- **NANCY KERRIGAN, two-time Olympic skating medalist**

- **JOAN LUNDEN, TV icon**

- **BILL MAHER, happily childless former host of *Politically Incorrect***

- **HOWIE MANDEL, funny Canadian**

- **JOAN RIVERS, perpetual hoot**

- **RAY ROMANO, whom everybody loves**

- **RICHIE SAMBORA, Bon Jovi guitarist and lucky apple of Heather Locklear's eye**

- **BOB SEAGREN, financial consultant and Olympic gold medalist**

- **WIL SHRINER, comedian**

- **TODD THICKE, brother and producer (*America's Funniest Home Videos*)**

- **MICHAEL TUCCI, actor/buddy**

- **VANNA WHITE, famous alphabet woman**

I apologize in advance for any offense taken by mothers who feel they are being joked about here . . . they are!

The transparent rationalization for concocting such sacrilege is that sharing a dose of gallows humor might provide a welcome break for any couple about to share the awesome prospect of childbirth. Otherwise, you may be in for nine months of PMS.

"IT SOUNDS CHEEKY!"

The tone here is deliberately chauvinistic, written with a *guy* attitude that fellas will understand because it's written in the male language, the way husbands speak and think when the girls aren't around. (Sorry, I meant *women*.)

(Note that I use *husbands* knowing full well that not all fathers are, including me. It's none of my business, and you may simply substitute *men* where necessary.) There are, after all, 14,000 pregnancy books for her and zero for him. OK, maybe one or two, but it's not enough. Someone has to tell the husbands what to do, and I've chosen me.

Our mission is to balance the scales, beginning with the inescapable disappointment men feel because we can never belong to *that club*. Only mothers can know what mothers know. Moms will tell you that childbirth hurts and they'd gladly switch places with you, but they really would not. I mean, to give forth a child from your womb . . . *wow*!!! The truth is we're jealous, ladies, and now you're going to pay.

How Men Have Babies is about male empowerment because the most important thing Dad can do is to assert himself *now*, expressing opinions with attitude and conviction even if you have no idea what you're talking about. There are a million important decisions to be made before and during pregnancy, and to be heard men must have the testosterone to stand up to their estrogen. I know this because my wife told me so.

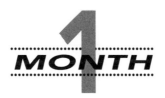

MONTH 1

KICKOFF!

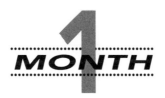**D**EAR JOURNAL:

This morning my wife said, "Let's start a family." "What a beautiful invitation!" I replied. "Right here on the breakfast table?"

There was a time when she would have laughed at that remark, but this was not it. The *family* conversation was one we both knew was coming since the early days of our courtship, when we discovered that one of the things we loved most about each other was our love of children. That common goal is right up there on the list of important things to know, alongside "Does she really like football?" and "Does he think it's funny to pass wind in front of my mother?"

Single men learn that some women can be courted to another level with talk about babies and that for these women the equivalent of "Talk dirty to me" is "Tell me about the baby we'll make." Apparently there are men on the singles circuit who lie and tease about such things for their own short-term gains, but these men are scoundrels and won't be reading this book anyway.

ARE YOU MAN ENOUGH?

When to "start trying" will become, at the right time, one of the most romantic and intimate conversations you'll ever have, a bonding highlight between you and the woman with whom you are planning to share a life-time of insecurity and paranoia. Subconsciously, even your wedding vows contained a hidden meaning: "I promise to love, honor, and torture in ways neither of us can yet imagine but I'm sure will somehow include kids." Nevertheless, you entered into matrimony with all the trust and confidence an airtight prenup can offer, and now you're preparing for the transition from couple to family!

STATISTIC

In 73 percent of marriages,
she decides when to start a family.

She may make it sound almost businesslike, like some irresistible investment, as though you might actually make a profit on this deal, reminding you that she is a goal-oriented person in constant need of a project. "How about repaving the driveway?" you suggest. "How about growing up?" she replies with no trace of irony. Your time has come.

HOW TO PREPARE FOR PARENTHOOD: ARE YOU SURE YOU'RE READY?

SOME FUN FROM THE INTERNET:

- THE MESS TEST. Smear peanut butter on the sofa and curtains. Now rub your hands in the wet flower bed and then on the walls. Place a fish stick behind the couch and leave it there all summer.

- DRESSING TEST. Obtain one large, unhappy live octopus. Stuff into a small net bag, making sure that all arms stay inside.

- FEEDING TEST. Obtain a large plastic milk jug. Fill halfway with water. Suspend from the ceiling with a cord. Start the jug swinging. Try to insert spoonfuls of soggy cereal such as Fruit Loops or Cheerios into the mouth of the jug while pretending to be an airplane. Now dump the contents of the jug on the floor.

- NIGHT TEST. Fill a small bag with 12 pounds of wet sand. At 8:00 P.M., begin to waltz and hum with the bag until 9:00 P.M. Lie down and get up again immediately. Sing every song you have ever heard. Fall asleep standing up, then make breakfast. Do this for five years. Look cheerful.

REASONS I AM NOT READY TO HAVE CHILDREN . . . BY BILL MAHER

- I already have girlfriends who call me "Daddy."

- My refrigerator door is covered with *my* artwork!

- They do say the darnedest things, but that's once in a blue moon, and in between it's a lot of drivel.

- I can't even keep my plants alive.

- It's hard enough to explain sex to your date.

- I know eventually they're going to grow up and write a book about what a lousy father I was.

- They get into the garbage and drink out of the toilet.

- If kids should be seen and not heard, why not just get some pictures of kids?

FROM RAY ROMANO

**When you wake up one day and say,
"You know what? I don't think
I ever need to sleep or have sex again,"
congratulations, you're ready to have children.**

FROM *EVERYTHING AND A KITE,*
PUBLISHED BY BANTAM BOOKS

MY BROTHER TODD SAYS . . .

It must be some kind of primitive drive to pass along our genes to future generations . . . because we all think we're so cool we'll be doing the world a big favor by throwing our personal pepper into the genetic soup bowl.

My biological clock was on alarm. We had friends who took years to get pregnant—according to one, "he wasn't shooting the good stuff"; he was "firing blanks." While I like to think of myself as somewhat of a marksman, how was I to know if my gun was loaded? What if it took a while? I didn't want my kid stepping out of diapers while I was stepping into them.

And so we declared insemination season officially open, and our sex life took on an added dimension—copulating with a purpose. Before you can say "morning sickness," we discovered we were as fertile as California farmland. As near as we can figure, fusion between egg and sperm occurred shortly after a James Taylor concert, where, incidentally, we had great seats.

When we first suspected, we rushed to get out the pregnancy kit, where she has to go on a little strip of paper. This is when I learned yet another difference between women and men: aim. But it was a bull's-eye!

I studied all the birth methods: Lamaze, Thompson, Bradley . . . underwater, home birth, midwife, bungee jumping, the White Water Rafting Childbirth Adventure.

Marybeth and I booked a tour of the hospital. Our group included a 50-year-old guy with a wife who couldn't have been more than 12 and a fellow with little English who wanted to know where he could get a sandwich.

I learned prenatal terminology like episiotomy. For those of you who don't know what that is, let me just say it involved the words, rectum, tearing, and incision. The next sound you hear will be me hitting the floor.

TODD THICKE, FATHER OF EVAN AND JILLIAN

THAT DESERVES A STANDING OVULATION!

For those who like a little science with their sex, the baby industry has invented the Home Ovulation Kit to tell you when your eggs are ready, much like the Early Bird Special at Denny's. "I'll have the whole wheat toast, sausage patty, and a healthy child with a chance at finding a place in the job market before I'm dead, please." With the Home Ovulation Kit a woman can identify the ripe dates in her fertility cycle. I was surprised to learn she needed help on this. I know when

I'm ovulating—I get frisky and transparently attentive—but sperm is always ready (it's a guy thing).
Apparently there are only a few hours of peak egg time,
however, and you must move quickly, or it's an omelet.

The problem with the Home Ovulation Kit is, what
if you're not at home when it happens? What if you're
at the neighbors' when all hell breaks loose? If she's
grocery shopping, the box boy could be in for the surprise of a lifetime. Okay, that was silly, and you're ready
for something important.

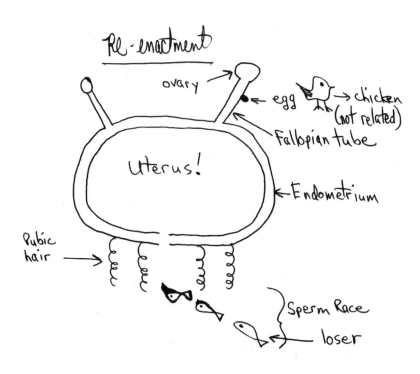

THE CONCEPT OF CONCEPTION

Pencils ready? Here's how it works. While you were watching the ball game, she was growing eggs in her ovaries. The uterus—impressed with the work the ovaries are doing—agrees to play along by forming a lining of tissue called the endometrium. This tissue is rich with blood, and around day 14 of the typical 28-day cycle, one of these eggs travels from the ovary into the fallopian tube in a nifty little maneuver called ovulation.

Even without your realizing that all of this terrific stuff was going on inside your loved one, you have noticed during the two-minute time-out that she is looking mighty fine. Remembering how much fun it is to sweat all over her, you smile, finish your beer and corn chips, and brush your teeth.

It is at this point that some men choke, aware that procreational sex is entirely different from recreational sex. Suddenly there is pressure. What if it's not a good sperm day? Relax! The old-fashioned approach to getting pregnant remains the most appealing to us traditionalists: love, romance, and prayer (her description). Mount up and let 'er rip! (his).

In the next 24 hours, if one of your 50 million sperm can successfully make the voyage into the fallopian tube, that sperm will have a chance to penetrate and fertilize the egg. (My favorite line from a comic to a heckler in the audience: "You mean to tell me that out of 50 million sperm, you were the winner?")

Sperm can live in the tube for up to five days, hoping to score. Consequently, lovemaking can take place before ovulation and still be effective because the sperm can wait in ambush for the unsuspecting egg.

The fertilized egg immediately closes its outer membrane to other sperm in an impressive gesture of commitment and fidelity. The egg begins dividing into a cluster of identical cells and exits the fallopian tube, making its way down to the uterus, where the cell cluster now divides in two. Half of that cluster attaches itself to the uterine wall and becomes the placenta, while the other half will become the fetus, which means young one. The miracle of life is in motion!

NOT DURING THE WORLD SERIES

One definition of *family planning* is to figure out the birth date before taking your shot (a sports phrase, to be sure). Let's admit it, fellas, we would rather not go through the delivery experience in the middle of the Patriots' title defense, a Stanley Cup overtime, or the Final Four of anything. Playoff babies are born with a chip on their shoulder, knowing Daddy wished they'd waited. Any input you have into the scheduling of your Great Adventure should include a preference that the big day come in the lacrosse or water polo season.

Aiming for Father's Day would be too precious to contemplate, and in my case, a mixed bag anyway. I've had some regrettable Father's Days, chief among them the one in 1984 when my first ex-wife chose to announce our impending divorce to the children. (I was happily married for 14 years; unfortunately, she was only happily married for 12.) It went something like, "Happy Father's Day and, oh, by the way . . . please don't live here anymore." I now celebrate Father's Day at my lawyer's house.

PMS STANDS FOR PREVIEW OF MOTHERHOOD—SIMPLE!

To forecast the delivery date, take the first day of her last menstrual period, subtract three calendar months, then add one week and project to next year. Remembering that pregnancy magnifies the emotions of menstruation, another way to calculate the due date is to take the first day of the last civil word she spoke, subtract the three kitchen appliances she threw at your head, and add one week from the night you slept on the sofa.

If your wife follows the soaps on TV, do not let her predict the date using soap math, where a woman stays pregnant for 14 months and then delivers a preemie. My 1970–1984 wife, Gloria Loring, was featured on *Days of Our Lives*, and when her character was expecting, she was also raped, plundered, pillaged, robbed, and shot. Most of you will have an easier pregnancy. After all that, amnesia was a welcome plot development.

HOUSTON, WE HAVE LIFTOFF!

If your wife chooses to announce her pregnancy in a candlelit room in the stockings you insisted she try on at Frederick's of Hollywood, enjoy it. This could be the last time in your young lives you see your beloved dressed like this. After getting focused on her upcoming role as mother, she may become Madonna—unfortunately not the pointy-bra one; I'm talking about the original.

CONGRATULATIONS!

Mission accomplished! Your wife is a sperm magnet, and you are the studman of the millennium! Kisses and hugs all around as she asks you to feel her stomach and you point out that she's been pregnant for only 20 minutes. She cries. It's starting.

TIP

As soon as you finish
jumping for joy,
call your favorite restaurant
for dinner reservations.

Make a point at the "Last Supper" to talk about sports and sex and any other hobby of interest to you, because this will be the last conversation for the next eight months that does not include the words uterus, mucus, or discharge.

CHOOSE YOUR IN-LAWS WELL

When you were courting your wife and, therefore, still on your best behavior in front of her parents, you probably spoke convincingly about your desire to be a dad. This often seals the deal since some in-laws want ten grandchildren. These in-laws are to be reprogrammed immediately or avoided at all costs. If you are shopping in the eight-kids-or-less line at the supermarket of life, and Grandma wonders "How many children will you have?" And you point out that the Chinese are allowed only one and she comes back with, "We're not Chinese." Keep moving your lips until something intelligent occurs to you.

Indulgent and generous are good qualities to look for in a grandparent, and you'll get a clue as to their GQ (grandparent quotient) by examining how they raised their daughter. If your wife was adored and pampered—no matter how deserving—you are no doubt paying the price now, but it will all even out in her parents' willingness to throw money and merchandise at their grandchild. And there's plenty to choose from. No one in America ever went broke inventing a new product to tighten your abs, lower your golf score, or spoil your kid. You take care of the safety crib, the safety car seat, the safety high chair . . . get Grandma and Grandpa thinking brand names right away, like Sega, Nike, Hilfiger, and Lexus.

Expect to be so head-over-heels over this child that you'll make comparisons to the Baby Jesus. Hint to the grandparents that frankincense and myrrh would make suitable gifts.

"LET'S TELL EVERYBODY! TOTAL STRANGERS! YOU, SIR, GUESS WHAT?!"

As soon as friends find out you're expecting, their first question will invariably be "What are you having?" The correct answer is (a) a nervous breakdown, (b) second thoughts, (c) flop sweat, or (d) we don't care as long as it's healthy. If you checked (d), you are politically correct and infallibly naive. Believe me, there's a lot more you can start wishing for. Make sure the grandparents' list doesn't stop at Hilfiger and myrrh!

Even as you spread the word, your dream is coming true and the fertilized egg continues to subdivide until he looks exactly the way you'd look if you were the size of a grain of rice. You can't see this division process, but you can hear it in phrases like "I feel nauseous" and "Don't touch me there." Things are happening that only women can understand. When you ask, "Honey, did you pay the phone bill?" and she answers, "Pardon me, but I only have two hands and I was busy implanting my ovum in the wall of my uterus," you know that you will be at a scientific disadvantage from this point on.

Some early signs of pregnancy include (a) enlarged breasts (See paragraph in Month 2 entitled "Things That Look Better than Ever but Can't Be Approached Because They're Tender"), (b) frequent urination (The Panama Canal doesn't pass this much water—carry a bedpan in the Jeep), (c) mood swings (Croatian politics is less volatile), and (d) fatigue (as in chronic syndrome).

SEX

Don't get excited; it's not what you're thinking. "Should we find out the sex of our baby in advance of the actual presentation of genitalia?" Many husbands want to be surprised at the moment of delivery. In one of God's cruel jokes, these guys are usually married to the women who need to know now.

If you've tried to influence the sex by conceiving at a certain time or in a particular position, good luck! Science is only now on the verge of separating chromosomes for specific gender selection.

*My father's scientific advice to me
involved penetration.
"If you want to have a boy,
you have to reach the liver!"*

TERRY BALAGIA, FATHER OF TERENCE,
SARAH, REBECCA, AND ADAM

HOW BEE GEES ARE BORN

After four boys, my wife and I were wondering if medical science had progressed to the point where we could guarantee a girl. Our doctor advised it was still hit-and-miss—much like the record business—but we could improve our chances with scientific procedures and injections when we returned from an upcoming road trip . . . if we could abstain for three months on tour. Easier said than done! The doctor never saw Linda looking the way she did one crazy night in Spain. The deed was done, and six months later we had our daughter. It turns out she couldn't wait either, and Alexandra was born a three-pound preemie. That's when we were most grateful for medical science and the fantastic job they do for the well-being of our little ones.

BARRY GIBB, FATHER OF STEVEN, MICHAEL,
ASHLEY, TRAVIS, AND ALEXANDRA

Discuss the "finding out what you're having" option early on, well before the information becomes available and your wife tries the old I-have-to-decorate-the-baby's-room excuse. Gina—that's Carter's mother's name—wanted the manger . . . er, nursery done in a theme so gender-specific that you wonder what those previous debates over equality, sexism, chauvinism, feminism, and other isms were all about. The decor would be pink or blue, rag dolls or airplanes, flowers or football players, period! I suggested a neutral environment like animals or clouds. That was the night I slept on the sofa naked with no blankets. Gina invoked study results from child psychologists who were convinced that early visual stimuli would influence the child's future. I humorously suggested a wallpaper design of 100-dollar bills. She suggested moving my sofa to the guest house. "How about a simple paint job and we'll let the baby's interests dictate the specifics as his play-time evolves?" I proffered ingenuously. "Child abuse!" she aggressed maternally. My feeling was that it would be at least two years before our baby started complaining about fabrics and color schemes, but, husbands, unless you are into sofas as your permanent sleeping vessel of choice, do not challenge her conviction that inappropriate wallpaper can indeed cause retardation. Pretend to agree that your baby will never learn to speak with ugly lamps in the room, and get on with your life.

In addition to the gender issue, there is another question about sex: "Can we please have some?" The answer you can expect is "Not as often, not so freely" and "Is that all you think about?" She may experience mixed feelings about sex, either despising the idea or abhorring it. "But honey, you've never looked more beautiful!" "It's the basketball breasts, isn't it? You may want to defuse this time bomb with a tongue-in-cheek response, your cheek being the only place, incidentally, where your tongue might be welcome for the remainder of this calendar year. Now is a good time to start reading yourself to sleep at night until we get to Month 7, when we'll discuss this further.

DATA

Toxoplasmosis is a parasitic disease that can harm the fetus. It is carried by cats, and you are advised to wash your hands thoroughly after handling litter boxes. Some things are just common sense, and personally, I didn't need to be given this advice. But they learn all about toxoplasmosis and a million other conditions ending in osis or itis from . . .

THAT CLUB YOU CAN'T BELONG TO

Earthwoman-Mother-Goddess-Queen of all living things and empress of the universe she allows us to inhabit international is a clandestine worldwide support network consisting of every woman who has ever borne a child. Mother-Goddess members live to play "Can You Top This?" with horror stories about their own pregnancies and birth experiences. Your wife will want to talk to every one of them. By phone. Your dime. The White House doesn't have a phone bill like the one you're going to see. Your spouse may actually look forward, rather ghoulishly you will think, to suffering every imaginable symptom and crisis her friends promised she would endure, filling out her calendar for the next eight months, prelogging each hoped-for headache, dizzy spell, and emotional breakdown.

By the time your baby is born, your Mother-Goddess will have suffered heartburn, constipation, hemorrhoids, and other plagues you thought only your golf buddies could have.

One reassuring thought is that as painful and terrifying as childbirth may sound, when it actually comes, it's worse! If childbirth proves anything, it is that God is not a woman or men would be having the babies. Why is it the best man for the job is usually a woman? (Don't think I've gone soft here. I may just be pandering. I included this passage in case your wife is reading over your shoulder.)

In these early weeks it will be a comforting display of empathy if you start reading some of those other books, impressing your loved one with tidbits like "the ovum can now be called an embryo." She may respond with things like "Don't bother me because a very primitive spinal cord and nervous system are developing in my amniotic sac." Once again, your day pales by comparison.

Soon the embryo resembles a tiny tadpole with a head, trunk, and tail that look suspiciously like her uncle Festus. Multiple tadpoles indicate another challenge altogether.

Dear Alan, How do you tell your husband you're having twins?

CYNTHIA, MINNEAPOLIS, MINNESOTA

Dear Cynthia, Thanks for your letter. How's the weather in Minneapolis? Are they ever going to have a winning NHL team there? Do you have relatives in Sweden? Do you like cheese? Sorry, that's Wisconsin. Anyway, the best way to tell your husband you're having twins is to: (a) tell him you won't need to have another baby next year, (b) call from the doctor's office and tell him you don't know who the father of the second one is, or (c) I'm not sure; let's ask Jeanette Onorati.

> I lay down on the examination chair while the nurse slathered that slimy goo all over the vast expanse that used to be my abdomen. (Why does that slimy goo have to be so cold?) She rolled that sonogram thing left, right, and center around my VW Beetle–size belly. When the doctor walked in, the nurse said, "Oh, dear. Look at this. Do you want to tell her, or shall I?" Thank God the doctor spoke quickly, so I didn't have time to imagine that the baby was missing limbs or that I wasn't pregnant at all, just immense.

"You're having twins."

What?! Suddenly twice as much was only half as exciting. With a 19-month-old boy/terror at home already, I asked the scary question: "Are they boys? Just tell me. I have to know."

"Well, unless these girls have penises, you'll be having two boys."

Needless to say, I didn't remember the drive back to work. I knew I'd better call Peter, which I believed to be the name of my husband. I started to leave a message on his answering machine when he came on the line. "Hey, sweetheart, can I call you right back? I'm on the john." I suggested he stay seated for the news . . . "We're going to have three boys!" He promptly had the quickest, loosest bowel movement in history.

JEANETTE ONORATI,
MOTHER OF SEBASTIAN, FRANCESCO, AND GIANCARLO

CHOOSE A BIRTH CLASS NOW!

If you were the class clown in grade school, birth class is the place for you. Fun tip: Bring one of those squeezable, hand-held fart machines to class. What a riot when the ladies do their leg lifts and you add a gas noise! The very people whose birth experience you have forever sullied will nonetheless never forget you.

Of all the things welcomed in birth class, be assured that this book will not be one of them. The sweet nurturing souls who turn their dens into schoolrooms and devote their lives to teaching others how to give birth have their own tried-and-true curriculum, and levity is not on the agenda.

One obvious value to these weekly meetings of couples with due dates near yours is that you will learn all the terminology necessary to communicate fluently with your expectantly beloved. It is important to understand, for instance, that the earlier-mentioned discharge is not simply a dishonorable thing that happens to naval officers after their harassment trial. You'll soon be familiar with nomenclature like contractions and pushing, and an air of maturity will creep into your vocabulary as you begin calling it a birth canal instead of the tacky synonyms you've been using since puberty. You'll learn that Braxton Hicks is not the wide receiver for the Green Bay Packers.

The most valuable benefit to her in birth class is the knowledge that she is not alone, that her fears and trepidations are universal, and that she will indeed survive and succeed. The instructor's den shelves are stocked with motivational books, and each week one thoughtful mom-to-be can be counted on to bring along some additional article or slogan of strength. My wife was given a sign reading "I am a strong, healthy woman fully capable of birthing and breast-feeding my baby."

I'm sure somewhere there's another sign that reads, "I am a 15-year-old peasant girl in medieval Uzbekistan whose uncle impregnated me before leaving for the Crusades. I will give birth in the fields between the cornrows with no husband, obstetrician, pediatrician, gynecologist, priest, midwife, labor coach, baby nurse, mother, shrink, or epidural, and I will finish harvesting my row of corn by sundown." Don't bring that one to class.

"OUR DOCTOR HATES YOU"

The additional value of your prenatal education is that at subsequent meetings with your gynecologist (yes, you now share this person), you will progress from being a faceless sex maniac who doesn't understand what she's going through to a certified copartner in creation. Your doctor will happily show you the ultrasound examination in which high-frequency soundwaves are bounced off the uterus, much like what happened at conception, when you bounced Celine Dion soundwaves off her uterus.

Before your first month is up, you will want to explore the choices available in birth methods, including modern options such as giving birth under water. This sounds fine if you're a seal, but many old-fashioned girls would rather give birth under anesthesia. Remember, they are anticipating the delivery of a football helmet through an area designed for a Ping-Pong ball. Gina had no intention of being a hero and called the hospital months in advance to put a hold on every drug available through the FDA and some that slip in past the border patrol.

Meanwhile, the doctor will remind you that she can't take pills and that the U.S. Surgeon General warns against excessive use of alcohol during pregnancy. Presumably, this advice is aimed at the mother, and there's nothing wrong with the husband getting completely laminated at regular intervals. Caffeine is understandably frowned upon; who needs to be more wired when you're already kept awake nights reading that your child will cost $400,000 over the next 18 years . . . tattoos and nipple rings not included?

No douching, no tampons, no saccharin, no nasal sprays, no aspirin, no Advil, no laxatives, no salt, therefore no lunch meats, no canned foods, no pork, no potato chips, no pretzels, no corn chips, no shellfish, no salad dressings, no diet drinks, no fried foods, no TV dinners, no cheese, no Chinese food, no saunas, no Jacuzzi, no skiing, no horseback riding, no scuba diving, no fun! No wonder she's miserable! A no-travel advisory is listed for the first trimester, but who cares? There's no place to go where they don't tempt you with all the above-mentioned no-no's. Thanks, Doc.

It was at the doctor's office that I learned one important statistic of particular relevance to me: 53 percent of all children who develop juvenile diabetes weighed over nine pounds at birth.

When my first son was born 24 years ago, either nobody knew or nobody told us that there might be a connection between birth weight and diabetes. Brennan weighed nine pounds, one ounce at birth and contracted the disease at the age of four. Scientists remain divided on their conclusions, but diabetes, once thought to be hereditary, has been reclassified as genetic, meaning that a certain genetic predisposition seems to be required for the onset. Diabetes itself is probably triggered by an as-yet-unidentified virus, and the role of birth weight remains under investigation. Until we know for certain, however, diligence about proper prenatal weight gain is important for reasons other than simply being able to fit into a sundress for an extra month.

HEY, I WANNA BE PREGNANT, TOO!

One of your roles in the birth loop will be that of the sobering realist while she reads parenting books with a decidedly more sentimental spin like *Cuddling Pumpkin Forever* and *Love Is a Big Poop*. You will at times have to rein her in with reminders that there will be pluses and minuses in raising this miracle: this living, breathing, sleep-altering, tantrum-throwing, vacation-busting, teacher-torturing, fender-bending miracle. (Check the "for better or worse" clause in your vows.) You will be the wet-blanket kill-joy buzz-buster who occasionally pees on her parade, but trust me, she'll thank you for it one day. Just not soon. For now, the die is cast, the plan is writ, the concept is embraced, and it is sinking in that creating a new person for the planet will be a very big deal. Deep in your heart you pray that you are emotionally and intellectually capable of influencing another human being in ways that will allow him to develop into something short of a serial ax murderer. (Please indulge my use of "him" when "her" could be substituted in your case. Hims are all I know.) The notion that a child may grow up in your image could be the most frightening thought of all, given the world's complete dissatisfaction with the way you turned out. Fortunately, men, you will not have to deal with this self-loathing by yourself, but rather, can rely on the expectant mother to readily join in loathing you as the months unfold.

OVERVIEW, BIG PICTURE, BOTTOM LINE, ETC.

By this point you might be asking, "What are his qualifications for writing a book on becoming a parent?"

- **The key qualification for writing an advice book on anything is to know absolutely nothing about the subject. That makes you curious.**

- **The best way to know nothing about parenting is to have children. I have three and can guarantee that every one is different and none of them knows the rules.**

- **One thing I do know is the Law of Heredity: (a) if your parents didn't have kids, the odds are you won't either; (b) all undesirable traits come from the other parent.**

Sixty-four percent of second-family fathers say they would parent much differently with a new child. It may sound somewhat biased to report that my two grown boys are perfect in every way—handsome, smart, lovable, honorable, industrious, and . . . well, you get the picture. I was a hands-on dad who missed nothing, loved everything, and tried anything, but the decades have seen some changes in the ways society expects us to parent, so this book will try to keep up-to-date by combining old experience and new thinking. You may be a thrilled, confused, intimidated, frightened first-time pregnant father. Maybe I can help.

PANEL

When my wife told me she was pregnant, we celebrated by having sex immediately (just to make sure).

CORBIN BERNSEN,
FATHER OF HENRY, ANGUS, OLIVER, AND FINLEY

We celebrated by arguing over how it happened.

MICHAEL TUCCI, FATHER OF KATE AND KELLY

We celebrated by getting married!

TERRY BALAGIA

FACTS

- A snail takes up to 12 hours to mate.

- A pig's orgasm lasts for 30 minutes. (But he smells so bad there's no second date.)

- Humans and dolphins are the only species that have sex for pleasure. (So the pig was doing it for money?)

- Some lions mate over 50 times a day. (That's not pleasure.)

- The male praying mantis cannot copulate while its head is attached to its body. The female initiates sex by ripping the male's head off. ("Honey, I'm home. What the . . .")

- What's the sexiest month? The average person's sexual vitality increases when the weather is nice. Women are more fertile in May and June, when the temperature is about 65 degrees.

- Sixty percent of all twin births nowadays are the result of in vitro fertilization.

- In President Theodore Roosevelt's second term of office, he told American women that limiting the size of their families was "criminal against the race."

- There are now more rats than people in the United States.

- What do you call couples who practice the rhythm method? Parents!

- Columbia University studies indicate that nearly 50 percent of all domestic fights start in the hour before dinner. Half of those end with someone's head in the microwave.

- If it's true that "guns are not the problem; people are the problem," then "marriage is not the problem; married people with guns are the problem."

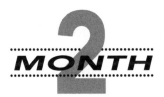

MONTH 2

BREASTS

I could have called this month "Nausea" or "Mood Swings," but this got your attention, didn't it? It is possible in the months after conception for a husband to feel left out of the loop. Don't worry; it will only last a lifetime. In terms of where her time, energy, and thought are being spent, expect to feel somewhat ignored and superfluous once the impact of your sperm donation kicks in. The reason you are feeling less important is that you are less important. The pop-to-be in the pecking order will rank somewhere after the baby, the mother, the doctor, the nutritionist, the birth class instructor, the nursery decorator, the workout guy, and the Krispy Kreme dealer. Deal with it.

The French have a particular name for this. (The French are very possessive when they're on to something and tend to claim it as their own. French cuisine, French toast, and that special way to kiss come to mind.)

The word *couver* means to hatch, and its derivative *couvade* means womb envy. All right, at this point you're probably snorting with milk coming out your nose at the notion you might ever suffer from a condition that implies you would like to have a womb. It has been said that little boys spend nine months in a womb and the rest of their lives trying to get back into one.

Womb envy can be defined as a reflexive jealousy that your wife is having an amazing experience you can never fully have yourself.

In primitive communities, men would show their empathy by puffing and grunting in a nearby hut as their wives gave birth. Dickensian man was known to puff and belch in a nearby pub as his wife struggled in labor and cursed the very name of the heathen beast who put her here. The enlightened husband will want to feel as much a part of her pregnancy as is physiologically possible but will ultimately be grateful for the parts he cannot experience.

Whether purposely or subconsciously, some fathers' empathy will extend so far as to mimic the mother's symptoms, including his own version of morning sickness and food cravings.

Other common expressions of couvade include:

- a sudden increased fascination with family history and distant relatives

- introspection about your relationship with your own father. Are your memories good ones, and do you want to be the kind of dad he was? How will you improve fatherhood as you've known it and be an even better parent to your child?

- an intensified awareness of your own mortality as you imagine how your health, your life, and your death will influence your offspring and shape their future

I was suddenly panicked and determined to reach every lifelong goal before this child was born.

JOEL RICE, FATHER OF HANNAH

- guilt . . . as you become aware of the difficult times your spouse is going through

- fear . . . including the fleeting notion that you might not be the biological father (Clearly this is a more obscure concern, and if the notion is any more than fleeting, get help!)

- jealousy . . . that you, the hunter/gatherer, center of the known universe, are suddenly not even the center of your immediate family but rather a peripheral player in the cast. This feeling may manifest itself in surprising ways, like trouble at work that draws attention to you and highlights the pressures you're dealing with. Some husbands have even had problems in the delivery room, such as a last-minute nosebleed, fainting, or "emergencies" that they will need to address heroically— like no gas in the car for the trip to the hospital.

There was recently a great wave of interest in an invention called the Empathy Belly, a pregnancy simulator that reproduces approximately 20 symptoms common to the mother's, including shortness of breath, increased blood pressure, and the need to pee every six to eight minutes. The Empathy Belly contains a "womb compartment" consisting of lead weights and eight pints of hot water. Far be it from me to try to influence what lengths you will go to toward exhibiting empathy for your loved one, but personally, I draw the line somewhere short of strapping a lead pumpkin to my groin. Call me a louse, but I guarantee that someday your therapy will be more expensive than mine if you need to spend hard-earned money on props to establish your sensitivity. If you must get in touch with your feminine side, shave your legs. Right now, your wife needs a man.

When you're feeling your most expendable, least necessary, more and more like the other four Jacksons, remind yourself that the average testicle is only 1½ inches long, ¾ of an inch in diameter, and weighs but half an ounce yet contains a third of a mile of tubes in which it produces those 50 million sperm cells in a single day and could, therefore, populate our entire continent in a week!!!

This is an empowering thought and, given what we now know about presidential behavior, may explain how George Washington got to be father of our country. Expect, however, that no matter their size, your balls will be busted this year.

I always get a kick out of the fact that during pregnancy men say "we" are pregnant. While they do share in the experience, I doubt there is anything men do that feels like this. My advice for husbands during "their" pregnancy is to try to be more understanding than they've ever been before . . . try to hold that thought for 40 years . . . then we'll be even!

One of the amazing things about pregnancy is the emotional range you experience. While I know there is scientific truth to the whole hormone thing, I think some of these mood swings are partly because we continue to get bombarded by fashion magazines that celebrate skinny women, and by comparison we feel bloated and distorted partly because we are bloated and distorted.

In addition to being overly understanding, one great service a "pregnant" husband could perform would be to intercept those magazines—especially the

Victoria's Secret catalogs—before they reach your wife, until she can measure up (or measure down) once again.

NANCY KERRIGAN, MOTHER OF MATTHEW

KNOW YOUR SPERM

The more you know about sperm, the more opportunities you'll find to include it in conversations you will otherwise be left out of. Be assured that your wife will seldom bring it up in social gatherings already enthralled with her ovary stories.

- **How fast do sperm swim? The answer is seven miles an hour, and you can't outrun the little suckers either, because they've got those tiny jet skis on the back. Reminder: a little sperm goes a long way.**

- **Now we can have our sperm frozen. It's tough enough to tell a kid he's adopted; how do you tell him he's defrosted?**

- **In vitro info: According to the Eastern Virginia Medical School in Norfolk, there is a great demand in test-tube circles for "educated" sperm from high-IQ donors. After all, who wants a Nitwit Sperm Bank? If you have a choice between the Einstein vial and the Curly, Larry, and Moe sample, who ya gonna go with?**

- **Opt for brains, looks, and athletic ability.
  "I'll take a cup of John Grisham and an
  ounce of Charlize Theron with a splash
  of Tiger Woods."**

Guys who are sterile are not necessarily impotent.
The pen works, but it's invisible ink. If you're reading
this book, presumably you've worked all this out.

> *My wife said the best thing
> about me having a low sperm count
> is that she didn't have to have sex with me
> to get pregnant.*
>
> TOM ARNOLD, FATHER OF NO ONE YET

MAN TALK

From the Internet, we get this further validation of
manhood, 20 reasons why it's great to be a guy.

1. **Bathroom lines are shorter.**

2. **You can open your own jars.**

3. **Your butt is never a factor in a job interview.**

4. **You don't have to curl up next to a hairy
   one every night.**

5. **All your orgasms are real.**

6. You can kill your own food.

7. If you're 34 and single, nobody notices.

8. Foreplay is optional.

9. Hot wax never comes near your pubic area.

10. You can sit with your knees apart no matter what you're wearing.

11. You have a nice relationship with your mother.

12. Not liking a person does not preclude having great sex with them.

13. There's always a game on somewhere.

14. *Sports Illustrated* Swimsuit Edition.

15–20. Being a father.

WHAT'S A DAD TO DO?

Recent studies show that dads spend 33 percent more time with their kids than their counterparts did 20 years ago. Including weekends, men today spend an average of two to three hours a day engaged with their young children.

Further studies show:

- **Dads push kids harder than mothers do.**

- **Dads use more complex language.**

- **Dads are tougher disciplinarians.**

- **Dads prepare a child for the real world.**

Growing up in the sixties, we still had a sense that the father's main role was as provider and roughhouser. The evidence of his love and involvement was obvious as he maintained a career and provided material advantages, such as a pleasant household, lots of toys, a good education, nice clothes, and an all-around nurturing environment of books, games, and people. The hands-on activities would include plenty of holding, cuddling, kissing, singing, talking, playing, wrestling, ball throwing, and feeding.

Noticeably absent was diaper changing. There's something about changing a diaper that for some time-honored reason, seems to define a good father in the eyes of the mother. Wiping a bottom, inhaling those fumes, and not throwing up becomes symbolic for all time in the eyes of the female parent—and God forbid we have not paid at least token dues in this area, or we'll be scarlet-lettered for a lifetime. Our shortcoming in the fecal cleanup department will be a sore spot invoked at our most vulnerable times in perpetuity. She may even stoop to reminding the adolescent child that Dad never changed a diaper, and before you know it, the whole family is in counseling.

HOW DO I CHANGE A DIAPER?

Carefully and at arm's length. It's important for husbands to know when to change a diaper. I figure every three weeks is about right. Some men actually enjoy changing diapers and doing late-night feedings. We must get to these men and talk sense into them before they ruin everything.

In fact, diaper duty—a.k.a. diaper doody—is one of the ways in which a contemporary father discovers the broad range of his capability.

FROM JOAN RIVERS

> Husbands are afraid to touch the child at first. The mother learns immediately that you can sling it over your shoulder and it will be just fine. Edgar never changed a diaper; he was very proud of that. My child flew through the air; he'd say, "she's wet" and toss her.
>
> JOAN RIVERS, MOTHER OF MELISSA

SCIENTIFICALLY SPEAKING . . .

Let's check on the baby in this second month. That cluster of cells is now the size of an orange seed and has become an embryo, which is defined as the *pre-fetal product of conception* up to the beginning of the third month. The orange seed's heart is no bigger than a sesame seed and has already started beating. The kidneys and liver are developing—presumably the size of a kidney seed and a liver seed—and there are dark spots where the eyes and nostrils will be, preferably below the forehead, between the ears.

Within weeks the embryo will have gone from the size of an orange seed to the size of a raisin, and her uterus will have grown to the size of a peach. You're still watching the ball game while a whole fruit salad is taking place.

As the new center of the universe, that raisin will now command more attention than any raisin since the beginning of raisins.

Your wife's blood is being diverted to the amniotic sac under the despotic control of this power-mad minigrape, which has now begun hollering commands at her entire body, mainly relating to nutrition. "Get me a supply of nutrients now. I want more protein *on the double*. Bring me oxygen, or you'll never work in this womb again!"

Just as the body responds to a bruise or a cut by sending extra blood and oxygen for the healing process, this raisin will be getting first-class service for the next seven months while the rest of her body flies coach. For that reason, Mom's hair may become more brittle and her skin a little dry or flaky, what with all the nurturing compounds like B12 heading for where the action is.

You can help by going to the corner store and buying products like body-moisturizing lanolin, aloe vera, and K-Y jelly (yes, *that* K-Y jelly). Wouldn't it be romantic to come home and say, "Honey, you look like you could use a little jelly?" You whip out your jelly dispenser with a big smile and—wham!—she bursts into tears. "Are you saying my skin is dry?" Once again, no good deed will go unpunished and if there are two ways to interpret any gesture, she will choose the one most likely to offend her, guaranteed.

In Breast Month, estrogen turns every one of her senses against you. You liked when she had a little estrogen because it provided a nice contrast to your testosterone. The combination of those two chemicals is, after all, what makes the world go 'round when they appear in equitable amounts, but when she's on estrogen overload, it's a mismatch. The dynamic is out of balance; the world is out of whack; it's a 5'10" rookie trying to post up against Shaquille O'Neal; it's not gonna happen; estrogen wins.

Estrogen is the world's most powerful drug and should be a banned substance. There oughtta be a law: the due traffic violation—Driving Under the Influence of Estrogen.

I've heard pregnant women say they should be allowed to drive in the car pool lane because they're driving for two. This theory has not been tested with the California Highway Patrol.

Estrogen is a steroid hormone that makes everything larger than life (this is not intended to be a Viagra joke, although I will stoop to those before we're done). In her world, the heat is hotter, the cold colder, the highs higher, and the lows lower than whale dung. Her body is producing hormones like Baskin Robbins produces ice cream—many flavors and varieties, each with a purpose. There's the instant-tears hormone, the what-if-I-have-stretch-marks-and-you-leave-me-for-another-woman hormone, the who-needs-you-anyway-because-me-and-the-baby-can-be-very-happy-together hormone, the where-did-you-go-you've-been-gone-20-minutes-oh-you-went-to-get-my-yogurt-I-forgot-oh-never-mind hormone, the I-wish-we-could-trade-places-for-one-day-and-you-could-feel-what-I'm-feeling hormone, the you're-the-most-wonderful-man-in-the-world-and-I'm-so-lucky-to-be-carrying-your-baby hormone. Expect this last one to be recessive and dormant for long stretches. (Note: The word stretch, as in mark, will cause an emotional reaction and must be used with caution until further notice.)

Get ready for the phenomenon known as morning sickness. For openers, morning sickness is a misnomer since it is not restricted to that day part, and you can expect projectile vomiting to occur at any time of the afternoon or evening. There is a fat chance your wife will go through her entire pregnancy without a single nauseated moment. There is a better chance that Elvis is a carpet salesman in Montana and that O.J. didn't do it.

Doctors advise that the following steps can be taken to avoid morning sickness: (a) avoid greasy foods; (b) eat a protein snack before going to bed; (c) don't get pregnant.

They tell you she'll have cravings. *They don't tell you* one of the things she'll be craving is your death. *They tell you* she'll want spicy foods. *They don't tell you* the salsa she wants is available only in the bandito territory of Mexico between 2:00 and 4:00 in the morning and not on Tuesdays, Thursday, or holidays.

There is some irony in the craving and vomiting cycle. How can you crave something one minute and spit it out the next? How can something so right be so wrong? Why does it have to hurt like this? When did this month become a country song?

MRS. SEAVER SAYS . . .

I was hungry . . . for very specific things. Not ice cream and pickles but peaches—all kinds of peaches. I ate peaches day and night, especially near the end. It is widely known in medical circles that too much fruit can cause digestive abnormalities, such as the buildup of surprising amounts of unpredictable gas. I made this embarrassing discovery the night before going into labor. I was in a bookstore following my (first) husband around when suddenly from my gargantuan body came—pardon the scientific term—a fart. It wasn't loud and didn't call attention to itself but was, nonetheless, an audible and fragrant passage of wind. The gentleman standing beside my husband shot him a disapproving look and quickly left for another aisle. One of the advantages of being a woman is we are never assumed to be the farters. Nearby, a number of patrons stood quietly perusing the merchandise, and it happened again. This time my husband looked at me in horror, and he was the one who left for another aisle. I followed, but by now I had started to laugh, and with each giggle came another gaseous emission. The image of a bloated farting pregnant woman hysterically chasing her husband through a bookstore was finally too hilarious to bear. I ran laughing out the door and into a crowd of people waiting for a bus. One final supersonic blast cleared the bus stop in seconds. Ashley was born the next day at 12:38 P.M. with a peaches-and-cream complexion—at the height of peach season.

JOANNA KERNS, MOTHER OF ASHLEY

"YOU STINK!"

Every scent will be painfully enhanced until it seems to come from the bowels of hell itself. You won't eat Italian because she hates the smell of noodles. She now hates the smell of the cologne she got you for Christmas, and if you wear it one more time, she'll hate you. Until further notice, you will go completely unscented into that cruel world each morning and become repulsive to the rest of civilized society.

You won't go to the movie theater because she hates the smell of upholstery. That was nothing compared to Gina's distaste for the smell of popcorn and for me at buying it. I am one of those guys who gets his popcorn buttered halfway up the container and then again when it's full. I usually instruct the concession attendant to pour on more butter than he ever thought possible . . . and then to double it. I sometimes threaten the vendor, staring at his ID badge and taking names if there's one kernel unbuttered. I then further horrify my cardiologist by grabbing a fistful of those stingy little salt packets and stuffing them into my pants pocket for the long movie ahead. Admittedly, the end result is a lapful of hot, greasy, salty, fake, dairy product smelling in its totality like open-heart surgery. (I'm making myself hungry just writing this.)

I would not have been unsympathetic had my wife simply turned to me and said, "Sweetie, can you hold that on the other side, away from me?" Instead, she began a gurgling, salivating sound that attracted my attention and that of the four rows in front. Her nose began to curl up, and her lips grimaced downward as her stomach contracted and her body lurched forward. Her arms flailed, one knocking the popcorn out of my lap on to the floor and the other grabbing my forearm to push me out of the chair with the bad-smelling upholstery.

After being dragged up the theater aisle and into the parking lot, I witnessed Gina's first emergency antisocial behavior. So uncontrollable was her nausea that she blew chunks on a Mercedes when a perfectly good Dodge was only a few feet away. You hate to see your loved one so miserable with you so powerless to help, but doctors tell us the correct behavior is to let time stand still and give her all the space she needs, no matter that the Mercedes owner may approach at any moment. Hold her tightly for physical stability, keep her head down, and stroke the back of her neck. If ice is available, apply that to the forehead or the back of the neck to normalize her temperature as she has no doubt shot up a couple of degrees. Use soothing, gentle words, and don't ask too many questions because it's difficult to toss cookies and make small talk at the same time.

Having redecorated the parking lot, we got in the car and proceeded home. Imagine my shock 15 minutes later when she had a craving for a Fat Burger. Is this some kind of perverse joke? "No," she replied, "it's a craving, and there's no explaining it, so take me to a Fat Burger or I'll kill you." This is the stuff of which dreams are made. Two people bonding, heaving, vandalizing, making death threats, and pigging out together.

There could be life forms on a far-off planet that have more heightened sensory awareness, but for now if you have body odor, bad breath, shampoo residue, navel plaque, stale washcloth stench, or ear wax aroma, she'll pick up on it from a hundred paces. You point out that your personal hygiene is as diligent as always, but her new and improved sinus function ranks right up there with technology's most sophisticated sonar devices and MRI techniques, neither of which can compare with her capacity to bust you if, God forbid, you even think about garlic in her zip code!

As mentioned earlier, this super sensitivity will not

be confined to her nostrils. She is experiencing every-thing for two and could probably out-perceive the entire Psychic Friends Network. (Are they still around? No? They should have seen it coming.) This would be a great time to take your wife to Las Vegas, sit her down at the blackjack table, and hope for a big enough score to offset some of the expenses that will frighten you in Month 4.

A WORD ABOUT PEEING

"I have to pee." You've heard this before at the most inconvenient times but never with this urgency and fre-quency. You already know that women are different, that men have bladders but women just have pipes with apparently no absorbency—pipes that need draining hourly, every 20 minutes if you're in a car or in a hurry. Now that she's pregnant, it's every 6 to 8 minutes. (An exaggeration. The truth? Every 45 minutes, compared to five or six times a day in nonpregnancy.)

THE GREAT TOILET SEAT FIASCO

Leaving the seat up is a new category of spousal abuse. I had been living as a bachelor with my two teenage boys, so we had a long history of vertical toilet seats in our house. Gina had us potty trained in about three months, however, by loudly slamming every

errant commode top she came across
message. For some women, their gre
is not by fire or drowning but by wa
middle of the night where she will sit down,
break her neck, and die. Personally, I'm amazed that
anyone would sit down without checking if there's a
seat there. A man would never think of squatting any-
place—in a restaurant, on a subway, certainly not on a
toilet—without assurance that there will be something
to catch his ass. The up-and- down problem was so
much pressure in pregnancy, I took the easy road and
left the seat down for nine months.

THINGS THAT LOOK BETTER THAN EVER BUT CAN'T BE TOUCHED BECAUSE THEY'RE TENDER

Your wife is going through more changes than
she's seen since puberty, which was probably the last
time she checked the mirror hourly for changes in her
physical appearance. Were her breasts bigger? Her hips?
Was her waist smaller? Would boys look at her differently? Would the school quarterback finally notice? Was
he still more interested in her friend Alicia? Why is your
wife thinking about this guy now that she's pregnant
with you?

As good as she feels about herself and her sense of
accomplishment, that's how bad she may feel about
who she once was. The svelte coed who could party all

night now worries if that playful, devil-may-care part of her personality will ever return. Or will she forever be the Mom? Will she be able to have them both, do it all, and be the Wonder Woman that a generation of feminists promised she could be?

> You gotta have fun with pregnancy, with the look . . . you gotta enjoy that time. That's what I told my wife. She was unhappy about being pregnant when she was naked, so I got creative. . . . Try this: if you put a feather duster in her butt, she'll look like Foghorn Leghorn. It's kinda neat. Actually, I can't imagine anybody else doing that. I'm sorry if I just painted a picture nobody wanted.
>
> **HOWIE MANDEL, FATHER OF JACKIE, ALEX, AND RILEY**

Expect her to panic when she feels she has no control over what's happening in her body, and be heroic by reminding her that everything will be fine when the baby's a month old because then she can return to work by day and have sex with you every night at her prenatal weight. Yeah, right!

Ironically, a donut the size of a truck tire will be the answer to many of her problems these days. It should be noted that the national cuisine of Canada is donuts. We have more donuts than pucks, and you can find a shop on every block: Tim Horton's Donuts, Country Style Donuts, City Style Donuts, Medium-Size-Town Style Donuts, Donuts 'R' Us, Donuts for Days, Dialing for Donuts. Next time you visit, take a look around and see if I'm lying.

ANOTHER REASON TO AVOID CHINESE FOOD

Some cravings must be discouraged because they're just too damn inconvenient. There is a delicacy in China called *hass mae*, a seasoning that translated into English means "sperm of the toad." Apparently this is tasty. There is no known documentation to explain who first discovered that sperm of the toad tasted good, but the gathering of this material is a cottage industry in China. Being a toad semen harvester looks good on a résumé because a prospective employer will conclude that this guy will do anything.

There is no telling what procedure is used to harvest the sperm of a toad. Presumably, you get them in a room with a Frog-of-the-Month pinup and harvest away. Do your pregnant Chinese friends a favor and turn them on to donuts.

SOMETHING IMPORTANT

One particular concern in this second month is the fact that approximately 20 percent of all pregnancies end in miscarriage, most of those during the first trimester. Many in your wife's circle will miscarry once before achieving a full-term, successful pregnancy the next time, and it would be wise to discuss this in the early stages so as to reduce the fear of the unknown. As disappointing and depressing as a miscarriage might be, it in no way precludes your getting pregnant again with a happier result.

It is advisable to think of pregnancy as a 12-month process and, at least 3 months before trying to conceive, have a checkup and make sure she's eating properly and avoiding alcohol and drugs.

The reasons for miscarriage are varied and include overwork, fatigue, undernourishment, anxiety, and stress—or some fluke of nature that simply results in the embryo not sticking to the uterine wall and, therefore, not getting the nutrition it needs, resulting in its atrophying, being too weak to hold on, and ultimately expelling itself. It hurts. It's sad and you'll cry, but it's not the end of the world, and with luck you'll have another chance.

Note to the Wife: Now that it's official, whatever you thought made you important before is less important than this. Wherever you go for these next 7 months, you will be center stage, as special as anyone can be. You have a glow, you are a magnet, you are Mother Earth, and your radiant circumstance will arouse the interest and curiosity of friends, family, and total strangers. You will feel so famous and scrutinized, you'll wonder where the paparazzi are. You'll be expecting photographers, reporters, and eyewitness news teams on your doorstep and behind every hedge. You are soon to give the performance of a lifetime, and in anticipation of that, the whole world is watching. Enjoy!

Wayne Gretzky's wife, Janet Jones, is an example of a total babe who became a total pregnant babe.

Janet was blossoming in her pregnancy when we did a weeklong house-sitting stint at, coincidentally, Alan's home in L.A. The most appealing thing about his house—other than the fact that he wasn't in it—was the second floor Jacuzzi, which overlooked the tennis and basketball court where Alan's teenage sons shot hoops. At 4:00 every afternoon, Janet, her stomach, and I would squeeze into the tub for a relaxing bubble bath. We ended with her toweling off in front of the mirror and both of us admiring her new body and assuming we had the privacy of a full-length, one-way window. By the end of the week, Janet had added a few dance steps from *A Chorus Line* to our ritual when we noticed the basketball game had grown from 5, to 10, now 20 players. It was only when I joined a game that I looked up at the second floor and confirmed that the window was in fact a two-way and the 4:00 bath had become a *Full Monty* floor show. Alan says that week was the one in which his sons discovered puberty.

WAYNE GRETZKY,
FATHER OF PAULINA, TREVOR, TY, AND TRAVIS

PANEL

The best advice for a pregnant husband would be to always remember . . .

Just say yes.

BOB SEAGREN, FATHER OF MIKA AND MCKENZIE

Lie about the size of her ass.

WIL SHRINER, FATHER OF NICHOLAS AND NATALIE

FACTS

- In pregnancy, the ovaries produce as much estrogen in a single day as a nonpregnant woman does in three years.

- What aroma best defines America? Forty percent of the population answered barbecue.

- The key to Sandra Bullock's heart is cheap men's cologne. Sandra says her Dad "used to wear Old Spice and Brut. Any boyfriend who wears something like it drives me crazy."

- When Rachel (Jennifer Aniston) was pregnant on *Friends*, the show's costumer was determined to keep her stylish. Her white blouse with oversized cuffs cost $98, the cropped jeans $110, and a string-tied T-shirt $52.

Brad Pitt wore a thong during this period. (I'm speculating.)

- **Mr. Average American:**
    - **stands 5'9" and weighs 172 pounds**
    - **makes love for an average of 10 minutes (even longer if he has a partner)**
    - **has sex with 5 to 10 partners in his lifetime**
    - **loses his virginity at 17, is married at 26**
    - **makes $30,000 a year**
    - **spent $450 on jewelry last year**
    - **drank 11 beers in the last 7 days**
    - **lives for 73 years**

I know I didn't say much about breasts, but there's more in Month 4.

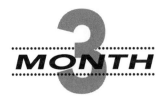

MONTH 3

DECISIONS

Scientifically speaking, your embryo has gradu-
ated from small fruit to medium-size shrimp,
two inches long and less than half an ounce. Already
the genitals as well as the other vital organs are beginning to form.

Your uterus (yes, it is now a three-way time-share
co-op) will be the size of a grapefruit before the third
month is over and Mom's nausea begins to wane and
her energy picks up—although she may not want to tell
you because sympathy is important and she doesn't
want to blow it by appearing too happy.

Most of the decisions you and your spouse have
had to make since you fell in love have been relatively
easy—what movie to see, what restaurant to try, what
outfit to wear.

This would be a good month in which to reminisce about your relationship: how you met, how you proposed, your wedding, the honeymoon, and anything else that will remind you why all this is happening. Plan a quiet evening browsing through photo albums and watching home videos to refocus on the sentiments that got you where you were before she said, "You stink!"

I met Gina when we cohosted the 1992 Miss World Pageant on the ABC network. She had been Miss World '91 and I had *never* been Mr. World, so already we had experiential discrepancies. (You've heard the pageant host say that "all women on this stage tonight are winners," and this is correct. The only difference is that one girl will get a date with Donald Trump and the other 49 will have nobody meeting them at the airport. One gets a job as an anchorwoman, and 49 end up behind the counter at the Big Gulp saying, "Want a lid on that, Festus?")

The omen at our wedding ceremony was a helicopter hovering overhead. We couldn't hear all the vows, so, apparently some of the promises didn't count. I got the "Do you take" part, but after that it's kind of fuzzy.

Once you enter into the married life, expect a few changes in your lifestyle. I didn't date as much, for one thing. A few surprises, too. You may learn she doesn't like football as much as she said and likes to sleep a lot. My wife thought she was marrying the perfect husband from *Growing Pains* and instead got the guy who throws his socks in a ball in the corner and makes weird and frightening sounds with his body.

Contrary to popular myth, people in Hollywood don't marry for money; they marry for love. They *divorce* for money. And you would expect marriages among the "beautiful people" to produce beautiful offspring but some showbiz children will be in for a cruel surprise. Two nice-looking people get married in Hollywood, neither one tells the other they both had nose jobs, and they give birth to a kid with a honker the size of the Baja Peninsula. They say, "Where did we go wrong?" It's not nice to fool Mother Nature. The kid gets a job sniffing shoes at the airport, and reindeer follow him home at Christmas. This is cruel parenting. But I digress . . . as expected. The point is to get each other in the mood to make the many important decisions required at this stage in the birth process.

CHOOSING AN OBSTETRICIAN

As a couple, give yourself this simple multiple-choice quiz:

DO WE WANT OUR DOCTOR TO BE . . .

a) **the old guy with the nice bedside manner?**

b) **the hot young woman fresh out of school with all the academic awards?**

c) **the hippy-dippy homeopathic have-your-baby-in-the-bathtub naturalist?**

d) the drunk whose license was revoked in the mid-eighties but who is starting all over again and offers the advantage of an empty waiting room, ample parking, and free rum-flavored candy?

By now it should be apparent that the phrase *multiple choice* is another misnomer. *Multiple choice* means your wife has not decided yet. Once she does, there is only one choice, and that is hers, and that's the way the world works, and you'd better get behind it.

WEREN'T YOU ON "ER?"

In Los Angeles, we have yet another category of medical practitioner to confuse the issue. This species is known as the *celebrity doctor*. His practice is based on a résumé not unlike an actor's and offers as his qualifications, not a row of degrees, but a collection of signed 8 x 10s like you'd see in a deli. If his gallery of publicity shots includes notably successful parents like Kirk Douglas (who begat Michael), Carl Reiner (who begat Rob), or Julio Iglesias (who sired that cute Latin singer), then he's probably a good choice. If his credentials say Menendez or Manson, keep looking.

When all is said and done, there is much to be said for that intangible *bedside manner.* My dad, the physician, figures he has to deduct two degrees from every temperature reading just to account for his own charm factor.

Growing up as I did in a medical home, I am often amused when a woman exclaims about her doctor as if she were his only patient. "He's so attentive, so nice, so considerate," they gush. The answer is simply that they sacrificed and studied for 6 to 10 grueling years, so most doctors did not choose their profession casually; their devotion to your well-being is genuine and comes as naturally to them as a Wednesday afternoon tee-time.

If you like a little homeopathy mixed in, you know that a calm, even disposition from your doctor can help the healing process. It sure can't hurt.

Stay away from a doctor you suspect has a one-size-fits-all approach to pregnant women. It's true; doctors see thousands in their careers, but one who has developed an assembly-line mentality would be a turn-off. One way to test would be to bring in a different wife to each appointment and see if he notices the difference. Have the confidence to approach your doctor as an employee—a very expensive employee, admittedly, but remember that he is working for you.

To establish a rapport, show up in a jacket and tie for your early appointments. Appearing in your jogging togs or a clown suit doesn't smack of the seriousness the medical profession looks for in making you a collaborator.

NOW PICK A PEDIATRICIAN

Reliable opinions and recommendations could come from your obstetrician, HMO, or local hospital. Pediatricians specialize in infant disease, but there are still some physicians around—especially in Canada— known as *family doctors* or *general practitioners,* who have the skill and training to take care of your newborn. These kindly anachronisms are on the endangered list and are likely to be old, but this could be a good thing. You might prefer a Jurassic doctor who's been in practice long enough to have seen it/done it and has plenty of hands-on experience.

Some parents take comfort in a doctor who's familiar with their family's medical history over the past 30 years. On the downside, there could be a lot of small talk about your uncle's gout while the clock is ticking and the time might be better spent discussing circumcision.

If it's a coin toss between him and the one who's fresh out of school with the latest science and procedures, you may choose based on location and availability. Is his office nearby? Does he or she rotate to different office locations? Can this doctor be reached by phone in case of an emergency? Schedule a get-acquainted interview to meet his other staff members. If they have that surly underpaid, overworked look, it might not be the right place for you. If the office staff appear skilled, friendly, and under control, they are (a) skilled, friendly, and under control, or (b) faking it. Rely on your instincts.

If the other parents in the waiting room look unshaven and smell bad, it may be a sign they've been waiting too long. You value a physician's punctuality, but, on the other hand, you may appreciate a doctor's willingness to spend a few extra minutes with his patient.

Does your pediatrician's office have a special play area for kids? Is there a separate entrance for children with contagious diseases? This is often used by visiting mothers who haven't had their hair done; are wearing no makeup; or now find the staff members unskilled, unfriendly, and out of control and don't want to deal with them.

While interviewing your pediatric prospects, discuss questions like breast-feeding and, yes, circumcision, and make sure your doctor shares your feelings about these delicate choices.

Is your doctor au courant with all the tests and monitoring tools you've read about? German scientist Wilhelm Roentgen discovered X-rays in 1895. In 1896, he discovered his pants were radioactive and he had glow-in-the-dark genitals. Much progress has been made since then in diagnostic technology for fetal wellness.

Check that your insurance plan and your pediatrician are compatible with one another. Managed care health plans are constantly changing, and a doctor who enlists with your plan one month may not be with it the next, leaving you with the difficult choice of dropping one or the other.

OUR DOCTORS ARE GOOD!

All kidding aside, let's get a few things straight about the excellence of our medical system and the ongoing progress we enjoy.

- **In 1952, polio killed more than 3,000 Americans, mostly children and teens. Not a single U.S. child has developed the disease since 1979.**

- **In the developing world, as many as one infant in four dies within its first year. India, South Africa, China, and Mexico—in that order—have tragic infant mortality rates. In the United States, Germany, and Japan, the rate is approximately 1 in 150, thanks largely to new medications that accelerate lung maturity in premature babies and neonatal intensive care.**

WHAT'S FESTUS DOING HERE?!

Start considering the cast of characters you'll invite to be present in the birth room. Assuming a hospital delivery, you will no doubt want to include a doctor. Your OB/GYN will offer an anesthetist in case you opt for an epidural anesthetic, and he will want to include a pediatric nurse to assist. Your birth class instructor may offer herself as a birth assistant or suggest a midwife from the class who is familiar with the course of study you and your wife undertook. She will be the one most likely to help you stay the course if your commitment is to resist the epidural (note the potential slugfest here with the anesthesiologist) and avoid the cesarean (note the potential gun play in this confrontation with the OB/GYN). International studies have indicated that the presence of a birth assistant has reduced the rate of cesareans, the length of labor, the use of pain medication, the need for forceps, and even requests for an epidural.

If you have decided on a birth assistant or midwife, be sure the hospital you've chosen allows her attendance, because some facilities won't permit them in the birthing room.

Also in attendance could be a group of curious onlookers and innocent bystanders, such as the mom's sister or best friend. My brother considered having laminated backstage passes printed up! What about your mothers? Has there ever been any competition, as in who gets to sit in the one cushy chair during 12 hours of labor? Who gets to hold the birth mom's hand while the other one fetches ice cubes? Who tends to talk too much while the other glowers and sulks because she's not the center of attention? Who gets to be called *Grandma* while the other settles for *Noo-nah* or whatever?

Somewhere in this mix should be the inclusion of the sperm donor. As the husband, you are entitled to be an integral part of the birth experience. You are the rock, the voice of reason and comfort. You will also be the soldier, the voice of authority who knows better than anyone your wife's wishes and choices as the options arise. You are expected to know her pain threshold, and if she has instructed you to help her resist drugs for as long as possible, you will be blamed if she folds too early. Your future will be even more miserable if you give her the drugs a moment too late!

As her chief support system, you will be the one charged with the ultimate decision: to videotape or not to videotape.

GET ME RON HOWARD!

Given your track record of being a fumbling dolt when it comes to operating the VCR and given the fact that you still can't figure out your car alarm and basically have no trace of electronic skills in your gene pool, you are a loathsome choice to video this once-in-his-lifetime moment. Blow this and you'll never rent a movie again without hearing how you botched the delivery taping.

For openers, talk about whether or not you really want to document this thing. There will be blood and some awkward angles with knees in the air and legs akimbo. Your wife may find herself in some positions that would challenge an Olympic gymnast. If your nephew is a film student and offers to shoot the event as part of his tribute to Stephen King, decline. It may be better to get it on tape and decide later if it should ever be viewed or simply burned. The point is, if you don't tape it, you may have regrets when your baby has his own baby in 35, 25, or (God forbid) 15 years.

Some couples would prefer to keep the birth experience as private as possible with only the doctor present. This is a romantic notion that will seem less important when labor peaks and she starts pushing and frankly couldn't care less if her graduating class showed up accompanied by the USC Marching Band and the eyewitness news team to shove a camera between her thighs.

SEX

Earlier I alluded to finding out the sex of your baby when that information is available. (See section entitled "Finding Out the Sex of Your Baby When That Information Is Available.")

FINDING OUT THE SEX OF YOUR BABY WHEN THAT INFORMATION IS AVAILABLE

More than a thousand years before the birth of Christ, the ancient Egyptians could ascertain whether a woman was pregnant by having her urinate daily on a bag of wheat and barley. If wheat grew, she was pregnant and would have a boy. If barley grew, she would have a girl. If neither grew, she was not pregnant and should find a toilet.

If you're curious as to the sex of your child and would care to experiment by having your wife tinkle in a bowl of Wheaties, be my guest. On the other hand, it is possible this method works only for Egyptians or mothers with a history of yeast.

AND BY THE SIXTH MONTH, ULTRASOUND CAN TELL YOU!

One couple actually filed a lawsuit against the hospital that told them they were having a boy when, in fact, it was a girl. What were they suing for? No penis? How welcome will the daughter feel when she finds out her parents were so unhappy they sued for malpractice? Don't let gender disappointment result in a dysfunctional daughter who will make you pay for the rest of your lives.

CHOOSING A NAME

*You would think we were
choosing the name for a new country!
This topic went on for nine months.*

MIKE HUTH, FATHER OF HANNAH

WHAT'S IN A NAME?

A Chuck is a Charles who didn't quite make it. On the other hand, a Richard is a Dick who did well.

Big Fat Tip on involving relatives in the choice of a name: Don't. Even in the most understanding of families, the name game can become a divisive tug-of-war. My sister Joanne had a classic case of name paralysis and consequently, unable to decide on a name, decided on 15 of them. She hogged every name in the New Testament plus all the kings and queens of England until all that was left for the rest of the family was Bucky Bob and Gunilla.

"HEY, GOAT FACE!"

In keeping with the Asian sense of humility, parents from those cultures were encouraged in previous centuries to downplay their public joy over a healthy baby for fear of making the neighbors and the spirits jealous. It was considered immodest to brag about your child's beauty, so parents would give kids lowly names like Goat Face, Buffalo Dung, and Wart Head. Presumably, this would keep them from shouting out at first-grade sign-ups or roll call.

Even in 20th-century America, there is legislation afoot to create some sort of government Bureau of Name Approval whose goal it would be to curb any overly creative parents who, in making their own statement to society, might call the child Feces Face. There are also cases of illiterate parents stuck for a name, who when required to put something on the birth certificate, might gaze around the hospital and arbitrarily pick an item off the food tray. The kid then becomes known as Lemonjello from Day One and is considered to be "a loner, quiet . . . keeps to himself mostly. We never saw him with explosives." Uh-oh! Surely, Condoleezza Rice was something her mother ate.

The following names are authentic, I'm told, and certainly fun to say.

- **Violet Organ**

- **Warren Peace**

- **Shanda Lear (of the Lear Jet Lears, honest!)**

- **Mary Louise Pantzaroff**

- **Miss Pinkey Dickey Dukes**

- **Positive Wasserman Johnson**

- **Virginia May Sweatt Strong**

FROM TODD THICKE

What do you do when your wife likes David or Carolyn and you like Rasputin and Thumbelina? We wanted the name to be unique but not trendy, sentimental but not corny, bold yet subtle with a taste of oak.

We tried out a few on the family. Reactions ranged from "That's interesting" and "How would you spell it?" to "No, really" and "Tell me you're kidding."

Someone suggested we wait for the baby to come out and see what name it looked like. That's how you end up with Red or Puffy.

MY KID'S A RAT!

When choosing names, be sure the initials don't spell out some unfortunate monogram. My second son's full name is Robin Alan Thicke . . . RAT! Sorry, Rob.

"HOW ABOUT . . . ??"

The most common choices for the millennium are listed on the following pages. Desperate for entertainment, you and your spouse can try to match the names with their popularity ranking and find the correct answers at the end of this month.

BOYS	GIRLS
Austin	Alexis
Brandon	Ashley
Christopher	Brianna
Jacob	Emily
Joshua	Hannah
Matthew	Kaitlyn
Michael	Madison
Nicholas	Samantha
Tyler	Sarah
Zachary	Taylor

Next, match the celebrity couple on the left with their child on the right. These answers are also at the end of this month; don't get them confused with the *popular* names or you'll have to start the quiz over.

(For some of these couples, the kid's name was apparently the last thing they agreed on. For extra fun, try to identify the couples who are still together.)

PARENTS	CHILD
Bruce Willis and Demi Moore	Speck
Woody Harrelson and Laura Louie	Sosie Ruth
Kevin Bacon and Kyra Sedgwick	Dakota Mayi
Don Johnson and Melanie Griffith	Ireland Eliesse
Sean Penn and Robin Wright	Indio
Alec Baldwin and Kim Basinger	Scout LaRue
John Mellencamp and Elaine Irwin	Chaia
Larry King and Alene Akins	Deni Montana
Robert Downey Jr. and Deborah Falconer	Hopper Jack
John Travolta and Kelly Preston	Jett

IT'S TACKY TO FAX

The happy pregnant couple must also decide on a birth announcement . . . and soon. Proper etiquette allows you to send announcements as late as six months after the blessed event, but it is bad form to wait so long that the card reads:

Dear Friends,

We are pleased to announce the birth of our daughter on August 13 (e.g., 1980).

P.S. We are proud of her graduation in business administration from Northwestern University and invite you to her wedding this coming May 4 (e.g., 2003).

For the tone of the announcement, many women choose a lofty, reverential sentiment commensurate with the miracle that has taken place, while many men prefer a lighter tone, more glib and comedic.

WIFE:
Oh yeah, but you're not the one who became a nervous wreck every time she had indigestion or a painful bowel movement, who's now lying here with swollen feet and stretched skin.

HUSBAND:
The celestial birth announcement will do just fine, darling.

CHOOSE YOUR TERMS

This would be a good time to decide on the terms you will use during pregnancy so as not to rub her the wrong way. (For "rubbing her the right way," see Month 5.) Some semantic tips from the Internet.

- Your wife will never *gain weight;* she will become a *metabolic underachiever.*

- It is not that she forgets to *shave her legs;* she merely has *temporary stubble reduction avoidance syndrome.*

- Her breasts will never sag but may lose their *vertical hold.*

- She will not shop too much, merely be susceptible to *child-rearing marketing ploys.*

- She did not *cut you off;* she simply *becomes horizontally inaccessible.* (She is not *cold* or *frigid*—merely *thermally* unresponsive.)

- She does not snore but could develop annoying nasal audibility.

- She will never be a negligent cook so much as terminally microwave dependent.

HELP!

It is during this period of fear and self-doubt that the two of you should talk about getting help—not just marriage counselors and psychiatrists but housekeepers, maids, baby-sitters, live-ins, cooks, pediatric nurses, and paramedics.

GET ME MARY POPPINS!

By 2005, over 10 million U.S. households will be using a maid, housekeeper, or professional cleaning service. Screen potential housekeepers in every possible way—past employers, police files, immigration officials—and be prepared to be shocked and amazed at what goes wrong in spite of your diligence.

The first housekeeper I ever hired burned the laundry and kept turning the vacuum on "blow" instead of "suck." I was frustrated at our language barrier, so I sent her to school where she learned English, found out how much she was making, and quit. When I explained that I'd like a refund on her tuition, she waited until I was out of town and invited her cousin and his friends over for a going-away party in my home. I am not a snob, but cousin Ernesto was in a street gang, and these people would not have been invited to a social function at my residence under normal circumstances . . . like if I still had one breath of life in me. They trashed my house by slitting the kitchen drapes with a knife, which surprised me only because I didn't think she knew where the kitchen was.

My next housekeeper turned out to be schizophrenic, which I hoped meant she'd get twice as much work done. Wrong. She simply had a dual identity: nanny by day; by night, lap dancer at a gentleman's club that featured a great deal of leather and chains. Chains get in the way when you're dusting. How could I have known from her job interview that when she said she was a strict disciplinarian she meant she wanted my boys to spank her? Mary Poppins she was not. I finally had to tell her I needed a different image around the house after she spent the night with a baseball team. A losing baseball team!

I finally found a housekeeper who was friendly to a fault. One night at about 3:00 A.M., she crawled into bed with me and my wife! Just lifted the covers, silently slithered in, and parked her whole program beside me. I'm not talking about Fifi the French maid here but a strong, substantial Haitian woman who looked like Karl Malone in a nightie.

Carla had always been affectionate but gave no indication of this type of employee bonding. The amazing part is that my wife, lying beside me, stayed fast asleep like a bear in a coma! I, on the other hand, perversely flattered but wide awake and terrified, tried not to react at all, pretending to be asleep, thinking maybe this was just a bad dream. If I'm lucky I've got food poisoning and I'll die. But Carla threw this superthigh over me in a leg lock that made my predicament difficult to ignore indefinitely. If a leg can suffocate, mine did. What do you do, call for the jaws of life? Try to guess her weight? I didn't want one of those middle-of-the-night confrontations where the lights go on and everybody gathers in the living room in bathrobes, hoping that someone can explain the ménage à maid phenomenon. Maybe she was tired from swimming the Channel. I figured this would be interesting enough when morning came and my wife woke up and . . . surprise! To my everlasting amazement, Gloria got up, went into that separate bathroom women insist on having (What's the secret there anyway? Is that where they hide the tennis pro?), performed her morning rituals, and left the room without noticing we had company. I've been ignored in bed before, but this was ridiculous! I finally mumbled something brilliant like "Carla, I hardly know you. All we've ever talked about is how I like my eggs, and right now mine are squashed!" It turned out she had developed a genuine delusionary psychosis in which she thought she was my wife. Soon after, my real wife started imagining she was not, and boom we were a statistic.

MORE SCIENCE

By the end of Decisions Month, you may call your embryo fetus, except in front of Festus, who likes the name Thula Mae and is now calling you Bonehead.

The fetus is swallowing and kicking, and the whoosh of its heartbeat can be heard through a special stethoscope. Do not be alarmed that the rapid fluttering you hear sounds like a hummingbird on acid.

PANEL

*One question to ask the doctor
is which of her new moods
are temporary and which ones
are permanent changes in her personality?*

ROBERT GANDARA, FATHER OF MAKENNA

FACTS

- What are the most common family names in the world today? Not Smith or Jones, but Chang and Wong.

- The ancient Egyptians changed clothing several times a day; people bathed in soda, and both men and women used perfumed oils and essences to smell nice and keep the skin from drying out. Body hair was considered unhygienic and was shaved by both sexes.

  Teething children were given fried mice to chew on to ease their pain. Migraines were cured by rubbing the aching part of the head with a fried fish head, thereby transferring the pain to the fish in what was known as transference.

  A common cure for blindness was to place the vitreous humor of a hog's eye in the patient's ear. A cure for shingles consisted of a frog burned in oil. Comparatively, peeing in your barley makes a lot of sense.

THE FESTUS FACTOR

- **Charles Darwin wed his cousin and spawned 10 children, including 4 brilliant scientists.**

- **Albert Einstein's second wife was his cousin.**

- **Queen Victoria married her cousin.**

- **In parts of Saudi Arabia 40 percent of all marriages are between first cousins.**

- **24 states ban the marriage of first cousins.**

- **Recent studies indicate that the risk of disorders like Cystic Fibrosis or congenital heart defects is only slightly higher among cousins.**

Still, you'll have a lot of explaining to do.

ANSWERS:

TOP TEN BOYS' AND GIRLS' NAMES IN THE NINETIES

BOYS	GIRLS
1. Michael	1. Kaitlyn
2. Jacob	2. Emily
3. Matthew	3. Sarah
4. Nicholas	4. Hannah
5. Joshua	5. Ashley
6. Christopher	6. Brianna
7. Brandon	7. Alexis
8. Austin	8. Samantha
9. Tyler	9. Taylor
10. Zachary	10. Madison

CELEBRITY PARENTS AND CHILDREN

PARENTS	CHILD
Bruce Willis and Demi Moore	Scout LaRue
Woody Harrelson and Laura Louie	Deni Montana
Kevin Bacon and Kyra Sedgwick	Sosie Ruth
Don Johnson and Melanie Griffith	Dakota Mayi
Sean Penn and Robin Wright	Hopper Jack
Alec Baldwin and Kim Basinger	Ireland Eliesse
John Mellencamp and Elaine Irwin	Speck
Larry King and Alene Akins	Chaia
Robert Downey Jr. and Deborah Falconer	Indio
John Travolta and Kelly Preston	Jett

That was fun, wasn't it?

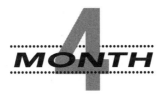

MONTH 4

MONEY

Seeing the first ultrasound is an unforgettable moment that will take your breath away. The doctor puts a palm-sized device on your wife's stomach that looks like it could measure the speed of a fastball. He'll move it around on her belly until you see what resembles a hurricane warning on the Weather Channel.

Swirling black-and-white images that will be completely indiscernible to you will excite your wife, who knows intuitively what all this means when she tearfully exclaims, "Oh, yes! There are the fingers and toes, and I see the heart beating." You want to cry along with her, but you don't know what the hell you're looking at. Now you swear it's one of those alien autopsy shots from the *Creepy News Gazette*. You can play along for a minute and say, "Oh, yes, there's his little kneecap," until the doctor points out that it's actually his skull and then bails you out with his assurance that the images become clearer as the fetus develops further, and you keep in touch via this video conferencing in the months to come. What a feeling to see that your baby is forming just the way he or she is supposed to and life is good!

Scientifically speaking, the fetus is about the size of a large goldfish but potentially much more attractive. You're still in the seafood phase, although hair and eyebrows are beginning to grow, clearly distinguishing him from an anchovy.

Blood tests can be performed to measure alpha-feto-protein (AFP), human chorionic gonadotropin (HCG), and estriol. Your wife will explain why to do this; I had my hands full with the spelling.

In this fourth month, your wife may experience quickening. This does not mean she's doing anything faster—quite the contrary. Quickening is the movement of the baby, and the onset of quickening will be a good date to note as it may help the doctor determine your due date more precisely. Yes, he's only been guessing 'til now.

By Money Month, most women need maternity clothes, preferably hand-me-downs from a friend or sister. (Estrogen is also known to be a leading cause of shopping.)

HOW TO ROB A BANK

At the 14th week in utero, your baby can smile and frown and is beginning to make sucking motions. That sucking sound you hear is coming from your wallet. Oprah doesn't make this kind of money. One question you may be asking about your own parental qualifications is whether or not you have enough savings. I don't care if you're Bill Gates, the answer is no. The economic impact of a child on your net worth is impossible to calculate, but assume that you will no longer have what they call "disposable income." Your financial solvency will forever be tied to this baby the way corn is tied to Idaho. Or maybe that's Iowa. I'm so full of baby info, I'm blanking on vegetables.

Hopefully, you have chosen a time in your life when you can afford to be pregnant, because opening escrow on a child is not for the faint of heart.

Adding to the challenge is that your wife, full of new life, is more giving and charitable than ever before. She feels blessed, she wants to share, and she will help anybody . . . the homeless, the helpless, the hopeless, the young and the reckless, the sugarless and the fat-free, the doofus and the penniless.

HER:
We have to give something back.

HIM:
We just got it! Can't we hold on to it for a while?

HER:
No.

True or false? No one can put a price tag on the joy of raising a child. False. It's $8,361,422.46. For the

price of an 18-year-old, you could have your own cus-
tomized 747, an NFL franchise, or a small country in
the Caribbean. What follows may be the most helpful
advice in the book since it gives you some idea where
you're going dollar wise with this goldfish.

In the first year of a baby's life, parents spend
$7,000 to $8,000, mostly on medical and child-care
costs. This is only the tip of a very pricey iceberg. Wait
until your seven-year-old needs dental work. Better yet,
don't wait! Start thinking about preventive measures
early on, like not putting the baby to sleep with a bottle of milk or juice. The residual liquid can cause tooth
decay, and you should try substituting water or gradu-
ally diluting the milk or juice until water is all that's left.

Setting up, furnishing, and accessorizing the nursery will cost more than $500, as will baby clothes and
hygiene items like diapers and wipes. Toys and books
can add another $500. If both spouses work, a child-
care center will cost an average of $100 to $200 a week.

Eighteen years from now, tuition and room and
board for a four-year college education could be
$200,000 and twice that much at a private school. A
car will surely be another million!

In previous civilizations, long before Kathie Lee
reformed the child labor force, couples would have
children to make money. More sons meant more tilling
of crops, unlike today when more sons means more
sowing of oats. There was precious little tilling around
the house when my boys were teenagers, and I never
got so much as one row of corn out of them. The

notion of children actually adding to the family coffers instead of decimating them seems laughable in the light of current costs, but there was a time when a man's prosperity was judged by the number of male offspring he sired. So valued was the addition of a boy that men often took concubines in the hopes of fathering a son. This sounds like a fine excuse to take a concubine but a questionable strategy for expanding one's net worth. Ancient societies, of course, could not have predicted gas money, auto insurance, beepers, CD players, and nose rings. A girl-child was so undervalued that some societies actually killed them, which would seem to be a little over-the-top no matter what you've heard about the problems of raising a daughter.

FACT:
A teenage girl spends so much time in front of the mirror, you have to wipe her reflection off before you use it. But boys are even worse.

Years down the road, you will wonder how a young man could possibly spend so much time in the bathroom and still end up looking so crummy, but every generation has its fashion statement, and grungy and disheveled can be just as expensive as scrubbed and preppy. If grunge happens to be in vogue when your baby turns 13, you may also be surprised to learn that smelling bad is part of the *look*. It wouldn't do to dress like a nineteenth century refugee from the Franco-Prussian War and smell like the Parfumerie at

Nordstrom's. Lest you assume that a casual, unkempt wardrobe would be cheap and durable, be assured that the Gap or someplace like it will have its finger on the pulse of any new fashion—it may even have helped create it—and will definitely have a Franco-Prussian department that honors most major credit cards.

"HONEY, WE'VE SHRUNK THE CASH!"

In pregnanthood, it is common for men to have anxiety about the family's finances. We would all like to live in two-income families where the Mr. Mom role is a viable alternative for hubby, but the truth is that even our enlightened society remains stuck on the image of men as hunter-gatherers, and if the cave needs more skins, Dad will feel the pressure first. Expectant fathers often find themselves working overtime or even taking a second job.

Studies show that some pregnant men play the lottery more intently or make higher-risk investments. Some may find themselves talking to friends about get-rich schemes that would have seemed folly only a year ago. It is important to be thinking about your family's financial security, but at the same time to be cautious about sales pitches from insurance agents and investment brokers who are trained to recognize your vulnerability in times of stress or transition. A Dad-to-Be is a prime target (i.e., sitting duck). Don't buy policies you don't need or make investments you can't control with money you don't have. Beware, be smart, and don't panic. The worst that can happen is that you will have a baby and become completely unemployable, lose your house and car, leave your wife and child roaming the streets in tattered clothes, living hand-to-mouth, while you stand barefoot at freeway off-ramps offering to shingle someone's roof in exchange for a jar of strained carrots. So you see, there's nothing to worry about.

GET RICH QUICK

Here are some tips from the top: long-term investment ideas from Edward White (father of Shelly, Alice, and Edward), senior partner at Edward White & Co., LLP, Certified Public Accountants:

- **Purchase an insurance policy on your life that guarantees a lump sum of tax-free money to your wife or children.**

- **Diversify your investments with stocks and mutual funds that perform well in a bull market and others that perform in a bear market.**

- **Work with professional money managers, and do not try to play the market alone. Use two companies and compare their performances quarterly. Exercise caution in listening to stock tips at cocktail parties.**

- **Fund a living trust to properly plan for your children's college education.**

- **Start saving today. A per-month savings plan of $250 may mature into a portfolio value of $100,000 to $150,000 in 15 to 20 years.**

On the subject of insurance coverage, be aware that if both parents work, each of you may be on a health plan, but many companies refuse to recognize duplicate coverage, and one policy will not necessarily pick up where the other left off. Be sure to notify your insurance company in writing about the baby and investigate your options.

Dear Insurance Carrier:

My wife just had a baby, and the guy who sold me this policy guaranteed that you would back me in this, so we are now partners. Congratulations! I want to have enough health and life insurance for my child's needs. That would seem to be $8,361,422.46. Regrettably, I have only $31 left (but the nursery looks great) and I would like to postpone paying for 18 years. When I bought this policy, you said you were "the company with a heart." Prove it.

Signed, Nervous Wreck

THINGS TO THINK ABOUT
IF THE WIFE HAS A JOB

In the prenatal period, most healthy women can work as long as they feel comfortable and their job is not too physically demanding, but do schedule your wife's maternity leave well in advance, especially if she is a bungee instructor or lap dancer.

Afterward, parental leave may pay 50 percent of her salary by qualifying for short-term disability. Help her with the following questions:

- **How much maternity leave do you have?**

- **How much of that is paid?**

- **Do you want to go back to work?**

- **How long can you afford not to work?**

- **How long can you stay away and still have a job to return to?**

- **How will you feel about coming home at night when your baby's already asleep?**

- **How will you feel about your baby getting its cuddling, feeding, songs, and games from another woman?**

- **How do you feel about your baby's first language being Spanish?**

- **On the other hand, what will you do all day as a full-time mother?**

This last question will answer itself fully within 24 hours of being back at home. The deeper question is "Will you miss the intellectual stimulation of that world outside your maternal sphere?" Ask yourself why you work in the first place. Money? Pride? Love of the work itself? Was it a job only you could do and your absence would send the Dow Jones plummeting or precipitate an emergency meeting of the UN Security Council? Will you miss conversations about subjects other than nursing, ear infections, and your husband's relentless libido?

Ponder this statistic: two-thirds of American parents are afraid they don't spend enough time with their children. This mind-set causes guilt, frustration, and stress and can make the time you do have with your kids more hyper and forced than it might otherwise be. These parents feel compelled to have an agenda for their family hours, and there seems to be less "hang time" for unstructured spontaneous activity.

Once we get over our own selfish concerns—and parents, by the way, are perfectly entitled to be selfish and put their lifestyle on a footing not far behind that of the child's—the big question for the ages is really this: What is the effect on the child when a mother works? In continuing the well-established theme of this book, there are no definitive answers, but informed consensus seems to be that the child will fare better if Mom believes she should be working for whatever reason. If and when Mom feels good about going back to work, her confidence and happiness will be obvious to the baby and you'll all be better for it.

Just after giving birth to my oldest daughter, Jamie, on July 4, 1980, I assumed the permanent role as host of *Good Morning America* next to David Hartman. I brought Jamie to work with me every day for the first seven months, since I was breast-feeding. She would sometimes get hungry before the show ended, and you know how that old mother-nature connection works. Responding to Jamie's schedule, my breast started leaking in my oh-so-pretty silk blouse! The hairdresser hurried to the set with a blow-dryer before a United States senator was seated for a talk on trickle down economics!

JOAN LUNDEN, MOTHER OF JAMIE, LINDSAY, AND SARAH

WHAT DID WE PAY FOR THIS BOOK?!

Take the time to make a list of the things you must buy, things that would be fun to buy, and the optional purchases you and your wife can fight about. What items simply prey on your insecurities? Your psychologist can sit this one out in favor of a bankruptcy consultant.

At that birth class, you can count on the other women to have a slew of prenatal products your wife hasn't heard about but won't want to miss. Start with the fetal phone, by which you can talk to your baby in the womb. (Get call waiting for twins.) Assume she will come home each week with some new "must-have" to go with the stretch mark lotion, maternity underwear, maternity bras, and lanolin cream that prepares the nipples for nursing (useless but fun to apply). (The other recommendation for nipple preparation is to harden them by lying topless in the sun. This has been known to cause traffic accidents and should not be practiced near a freeway. Breasts, incidentally, are an industry unto themselves—the pump is a hoot—and supporting this industry will please those men who've spent their lives fascinated with these body parts.

For bedtime, she'll want that two-sided comfort pillow that supports her stomach and prevents rolling over to a position from which she cannot return. Rolling on your side is the pregnant woman's version of "I've fallen and I can't get up."

Your beloved may hear from a rich friend that group exercise classes would no longer cut it and the only way to properly condition her body would be with a personal trainer. As part of this month on Embryonic Economic Enlightenment, you should know that an aerobics class costs $15 and a personal trainer runs $75 an hour. She's your wife, and it's your baby, and you may decide they're worth it.

HIM:
But honey, we bought $3,000 worth of gym equipment last year, and you were perfectly happy. What's the problem?

HER:
Do you want me to hurt myself?

PERSONAL TRAINER:
Hi, my name's Rudy, and I'll be here every morning. Should I stay in the guest room or just have a key?

Fortunately, you don't have to incur all of these expenses immediately. You still have time to save up, get a part-time job, start your loan application, or, as suggested, rob a bank. Statistics show you have a better chance of pulling a successful heist on a convenience store than you do a savings and loan, although the take might be somewhat less. A wiser choice would be to knock over a toy store or maternity shop since those people now have all our money.

THE VAGINA MONOLOGUES

In Saskatchewan, also known as the "Regina Monologues", a vaginal hospital birth costs about $7,000 less than a cesarean ($3,000 vs. $10,000), so please use the vagina wherever possible. Neither of these figures includes the doctor's fee.

TROLLING FOR GIFTS

There are some positive, preemptive steps you can take to cover the cash flow. Milk the baby shower for all it's worth by registering at stores at which your friends should shop for gifts. Be sure to make a list of all the things you'll need after the baby's born and invite people who can afford this stuff. Review your wedding invitation list and eliminate the cheapskates who didn't get you anything good.

CHILD-PROOFING YOUR HOUSE

This is a no-brainer, totally necessary, with no option or alternative. Your household and lifestyle must be examined to ensure maximum safety for the newborn. Obviously, your residence has to become more child-proof as the baby gains physical skills and more capacity for mayhem, so address those expenses now, before getting the fetal phone and the roll-over pillow.

The other purpose of the child-proofing industry is to frighten you into thinking that your home is the *Nightmare on Elm Street* and everything you own is a potential baby killer. In the old days, we worried about things like kids sticking their heads in the oven or running out in front of the ice-cream truck. Now it's drive-by shootings and the fatal possibilities of everything from an air bag to an undercooked burger. Admittedly, that light socket 12 feet in the air could hurt your six-month-old if he shinnies up there for the purpose of sticking his Swiss Army knife into the live electrical outlet. The probability of this taking place ranks somewhere up there with your winning the lottery twice.

The scare-mongers can be a little dramatic. A child-proofing company came and put a padlock on my sweat socks. They have a kill switch on my electric toothbrush, and a motion detector goes off when the dog farts. The things I used to look at, loaf on, play with, read, and collect are now covered in plastic. Artifacts I hand-carried from the jungles of Africa have been sprayed with Lysol and put in plastic cubicles.

At the age of four months, your child will exist for the sole purpose of putting the entire world in his mouth. He will want to swallow everything in his universe, no matter how big or foul tasting. Pocket change is an infant favorite and is especially inconvenient because you may need those quarters to park at the hospital when your toddler gets your Rolex lodged in his esophagus. To paraphrase the popular spiritual:

> **He's got the whole world in his mouth.**
>
> **He's got the little bitty earrings in his mouth.**
>
> **He's got the little bitty cuff links in his mouth.**
>
> **He's got the teensy-weensy thumbtacks in his mouth.**
>
> **He's got the whole world in his mouth.**

HOW DO YOU SPELL CPR?

Take a class in infant emergency paramedic procedures. For more information contact the American Society of Pediatric Rescue. Do it now! (Go on, I'll wait.)

Keep in mind that there is no substitute for parental supervision and everything in the house can indeed be dangerous in the hands of a child. He will break, smash, crush, crunch, fold, spindle, and mutilate materials developed by NASA to withstand any force or impact. This material may be effective in the path of an oncoming asteroid, but it is no match for a two-year-old.

REMODELING

Once you're into child-proofing, it's one hazardously small step to the next level: screwing up a perfectly good home. To a rock star, remodel means "date another model." To a husband, remodel means "paint the nursery." To a wife, it means "convert your TV den into a playroom, enclose the patio as a breakfast nook, and tear down the living room walls to add a guest room for my mother." Proceed with prudence if you're planning any structural changes in this already-busy period before the arrival.

The last time I hired a contractor, my bathtub ran only cold water. The only hot water in my bathroom was in the toilet. Did you hear me? My commode flushed hot water! No thinking person wants to start his day by pushing down on the handle and finding his butt in a steam cooker.

And this guy took forever to ruin my house. The first room you should have your contractor finish is the guesthouse, because that's where he'll be living for the next three years. Doesn't it amaze you that someone else can build 9,000 apartment units down the street in less time than it takes your guy to finish the kitchen? "Oh, you want a kitchen with a roof? You should have said something. That's another $2 million."

"How come it takes so long?" I asked. "Paperwork," he says. That's where the name contractor comes from. They don't build; they write contracts. "Maybe next time you come over you could bring a hammer instead of a pen."

After eight months we were halfway through the job and all the way through my patience when suddenly my contractor declared bankruptcy! How he could be bankrupt after what he charged me, I'll never know, but his legal defense was to prove his incompetence, which he did by showing Polaroids of my house.

Then he tried to blame the monstrosity on me, saying I was indecisive. So I decided to kill him (legally speaking, offing a contractor qualifies as justifiable homicide) or at least render him useless and unrecognizable, like he did to my house. Finally, the judge said, "You call that a roof? You're a nut. Go free!"

It turns out this guy had a drinking problem, so the judge sent him to rehab, where they had 12 steps (9 more than my staircase!).

MORAL:
Never choose a contractor
by watching AMERICA'S MOST WANTED.

Worse than a contractor is a decorator. I am embarrassed to admit that the remodeling for the arrival of my second son included a carpet electrically wired with thousands of tiny lightbulbs that twinkled on and off at night. I was afraid the dog was going to wet the rug and fry himself. As a man with a carpet too expensive to walk on and a toilet too hot to sit on, let me advise:

- **Remodeling can be dangerous. Don't try it at home.**

- **Make it simple and quick—there's a baby coming!**

BUDGET NOW!

The cash drain escalates about five months into baby's life, when you enroll in Gymboree, Mommy and Me, Kid Yoga, Friends of Barney, and any number of activity groups designed to get your child interacting socially with others and afford Mom an opportunity to get out of the house. At an average of $10 a class, you could spend $200 a month on activities for a tyke whose idea of coordination is to burp and crap simultaneously. Nevertheless, these groups provide an hour's distraction at a cheaper rate than the psychiatrist you've been resisting and a chance to compare your child with others in his peer group. Is he faster? Slower? Smarter? Dumber? Cuter? Sweeter?

The deeper purpose of mommy groups is to let your wife compare her postnatal weight with that of other women. If you, the husband, find yourself conspicuously not invited to these gatherings, chances are the class is full of supermodel types who have intimidated the hell out of your loved one. You may be perfectly happy with her postpartum physical condition, but your wife could become self-conscious about the rate at which she is not losing weight. Keep quiet on this one if you know what's good for you.

IS IT CHEAPER IF HE'S STUPID?

Use the play group as an exercise in preparing for the real horror of enrolling him in school. If you choose a private school education for your child, plan on beginning the sign-up procedure by age two. If you're lucky, you'll have him in preschool by the age of three so he'll be a pre-school post-grad by age four and they'll accept him into kindergarten by age five to prep him for first grade by age six. . . and so on.

Friends will happily offer you opinions on the best schools, and you'll soon find yourself soliciting their sponsorship as you begin kissing up to the school board. You'll be astounded at the competition among parents trying to get their children into a school that, if truth be told, is part of a system that places the United States no higher than 16th in the world in math and verbal skills. All this for only $12,000 a year for a five-year-old! What must it cost in Sweden, where kids can actually do addition without a calculator and use a verb and noun in the same sentence?

School waiting lists will seem completely premature when you're still negotiating the cloud painting for the nursery, but . . .

Your friends are right: you can never be too rich, too thin, or too early to register for preschool. In fact, having your child accepted can become the great ambition in your life as you scramble tooth and nail over Gymboree parents who might be perfectly nice people in any other environment but who now stand between your baby and a good education. It's like the closing scenes of *Titanic* in which a handful of the doomed fight for that last gasp of air before being swallowed by the cold, unfeeling sea.

Before your next child, you'll know to register for preschool as soon as you stop taking the pill. Clearly the leverage in this process belongs to the school itself, and you are but a pawn, a player, a statistic in a seller's market in which they hold all the cards. Nevertheless, you are entitled to reflect on these questions:

- **At what age do I want my child in preschool? Two-year-olds might be better off in play groups or day care. Your pediatrician will tell you that three years is a good age for preschool because they are more able to learn, are more independent, and can dress and feed themselves. They have mastered key bathroom skills and are ready for social interaction and sharing. Decide between programs that are child centered and those that are agenda centered.**

- **Is there a good child-teacher ratio? Be sure your child will get specific attention and develop at his or her own pace, according** to the child's own interests in art, sports, and games.

- **What is the preschool's orientation? Academic? Religious? Athletic? Artistic?**

- **What are the teachers' qualifications? If the teachers are 15 years old and come to school with their own parole officers, that's a bad sign.**

- **Do they offer flexible scheduling that might fit your own needs? That is, are they open 24 hours a day, and can the kids live there?**

- **Does the school encourage parental involvement? Other than inviting you to buy an ad in the yearbook, pay for a booth at the picnic, and donate to the building fund?**

- **What are the other kids and parents like? Are they all rich? Are we going to start the slippery slope, the never-ending spiral of competition to keep up with the Joneses and their expensive toys, birthday parties, and designer clothes?**

It is for these reasons that parenting in Beverly Hills can be a problem on a par with mudslides, earthquakes, fires, pestilence, car chases, and reruns. It's considered child abuse if your kid's birthday party isn't catered. Your six-year-old is an outcast if she doesn't have a sitcom deal. To avoid the pressure of materialism, never let your child play with a kid named Getty.

MORE ABOUT THE QUALITY OF EDUCATION

Years ago, when you drove by a school and saw a sign reading "Slow Children," it was a traffic warning; now it's a comment on our times.

How many Americans have high school diplomas? Eighty-two percent, but half can't read them, and ten percent try to color them in.

What standard should be used in school to determine literacy? How 'bout familiarity with the alphabet? (Those applying for athletic scholarships must know 24 of the 26 letters, although in no particular order.)

Do SAT exams discriminate against certain people? Yes . . . the ones who don't know the answers.

A few things to remember for those SATs:

1. **There's never been a pope named Scooter.**

2. **The capital of Zimbabwe is not Oingo Boingo.**

3. **Never walk into an exam complaining, "I couldn't study last night; the bar was too noisy."**

Take comfort in the fact that you are your child's primary learning source, but start on Day One or your kid's first report card could have more Fs than a Chris Rock monologue.

PANEL

The stupidest thing we bought during our pregnancy was . . .

the "Mercedes" of strollers because the store told us how much the baby would love it.

ROBERT GANDARA

condoms!

WIL SHRINER

a crib. I calmly told her that she was only three months pregnant and we had time to find one. Beth screamed, "What if the baby is early and the store is out of cribs and they have to order one and it gets put on back order and our baby has to sleep in a dresser drawer because we don't have a crib?" We got a crib.

MIKE HUTH

FACTS

- In 2010, a dollar will be worth approximately 60 cents.

- What the rich say they'd pay for . . .
  - A place in heaven: $640,000
  - True love: $487,000
  - Intellect: $407,000

- Talent: $285,000
- Youth: $259,000
- Beauty: $83,000
- Being President: $55,000

- **Average workweek in 1900: 10 hours per day, six days a week.**

- **Average weekly wage of a male stenographer in 1900: $10.**

- **Average weekly wage of a woman in 1900: $2.50.**

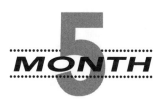

MONTH 5

BIRTH CLASS

*T*he car made its way deliberately down the quiet, oak-lined streets of the suburban bedroom community; his hands gripped the wheel with determination; his eyes fixed on the silent gray road that would lead them to the promised land. Traffic signs were perfunctory stops, faint tokens of obedience from a man afraid that too long a hesitation would give voice to her uncertainty.

She could taste her own breath, hot with expectation as they inched along, connected in a way that soul mates need not speak. Now on the appointed avenue, their eyes darted furtively among the street signs, inspecting house numbers until there was no mistaking the unobtrusive bungalow, surrounded as it was by a gaggle of family wagons, each having delivered its pair of disciples come to hear the Word, that they might be confident and calm for the journey. Too emotional to look her in the eye lest he belie the facade of strength and authority he sought to project, he opened the passenger door and gently proffered his hand for the steadiness and comfort only he could give.

Through the window, in the den, strangers introduced themselves in the short, choppy handshakes of forced familiarity that sought to break the ice in this sanctum of awkward anticipation.

He let himself in to stand firmly in place until all eyes were on him, then gestured back toward the door with one hand as if to create a threshold across which his pregnant angel could now pass. Seizing the moment, his voice reverberated in a hopeful bravado that let the group know and feel him immediately. "Hi, folks! So this is Girth Class!" Eight women, as if in one motion and without hesitation, reached into their handbags, pulled out their guns, and shot him between the eyes, blowing his brains out.

"Honey, wake up. It's just a dream!" Reluctantly, I told Gina of my nightmare about the impression I was afraid I'd make when we attended our first birth class and assured her I had learned that valuable lesson from the fart machine in Month 1: when meeting your coparents-to-be, don't lead with a joke. They won't think it's funny. They won't think anything is funny. They're skittish and taking this birthing stuff very seriously. Not that it's not the most important thing you'll ever do, but can't we all just learn to get along? Can't we lighten the load and cut the tension with just enough levity to make it the celebration we imagined childbirth would be? The answer again is "No. It's not funny. We're all scared. Don't try to make us laugh, or we'll hurt you."

You are at a stage where you make the turn from the nurturing (how to massage her thighs) to the frightening (how to deliver your baby in an emergency). You are about to meet the people with whom you'll be discussing the behavior of your wife's uterus and learning more about theirs than you ever cared to know. Soon you will be rolling around on the floor together, each of you rubbing your spouse's buttocks in the kind of group scene you thought went out with the Free Love Boogie Nights of the seventies.

More dauntingly, you will learn how to grab your baby's head when it first clears the birth canal, twisting it to the side and clearing the baby's breathing passage. Geez! Don't some people spend years in medical school for that? I saw this on "ER," and it took 6 doctors! Even George Clooney looked nervous. How am I supposed to know what to do in 12 easy lessons? It has long been my opinion that certain chores should be left to highly trained professionals, consistent with the "Don't try this at home" philosophy. For instance, I've never understood the appeal of learning to fly your own airplane. If I'm going to be five miles off the ground, I want to return to earth in a logical, well-thought-out manner, arranged by someone who studied this procedure and has a checklist of maneuvers and safeguards.

Thinking ahead, I have the same feeling about vasectomies. If there's a Home Vasectomy Kit, leave it off my gift list. I want to place my valuables in the hands of a seasoned pro who will do his job with precision and tenderness. I want to apply this cautious approach to childbirth and yet have found myself in a classroom in which half the students are perfectly willing to go it alone at home without benefit of the centuries of medical progress we now have at our fingertips. More power to them. I respect their choices and admire these people. I just don't happen to be one of them.

The first thing you will notice about your instructor is that her blouse is wrinkled and her sweatpants have ketchup stains on them, as if she might have starred in one of those disturbing Carl's Jr. commercials where the condiments end up in your lap because you can't get them all in your mouth. The assumption here is that she cares much less about her own appearance than the children she has unselfishly chosen to raise.

Her indulgent, caring manner is so genuine it makes you feel guilty for your own cynical, shallow posture, which, in truth, only masks your fear.

She looks harmless, but remember, she is your wife's co-conspirator on the grassy knoll of childbirth, and when any choice comes up for a vote, it's their two against your one, no Florida recount.

She begins by telling you to find a comfortable seat. The women choose padded mats on the floor, and the men who don't get it yet gravitate to the sofa. Our instructor, Mrs. Helfond, then cheerily announced she would take a photograph to memorialize the occasion. "Mr. Thicke, why don't you get down on the floor with the others so I can get you all in?"

Class began with Mrs. Helfond inviting us to go around the room telling our names, what we did for a living, and the official start date of our pregnancy. This is where I learned that the first day of bleeding in her last menstrual period is considered the official date because it's easier to identify than the date of conception. All the other fathers knew the bleeding day. Why am I the only guy who remembers the date of conception? Has it been that rare? Are they all getting more than me? Odd man out again.

Maybe we should take a step back in time and make sure that you've chosen the right birth class. Who recommended this Mrs. Helfond, anyway? The best endorsement is usually word-of-mouth from one of your wife's friends who has recently given birth and raves about her instructor.

> *We had this young, pretty nurse*
> *who would sit in front of the dads*
> *and spread her legs wide open*
> *and rub herself to demonstrate the massage.*
> *Needless to say, I never missed a class.*
>
> TERRY BALAGIA

I think you missed the point, Terry.

In class, you will find the overall level of teacher-pupil acceptance to be more than what you got in high school. There is little likelihood you will be told to pipe down or stand in the hall, and you would have to be a real jerk to actually fail this class, given the importance of the material and the saintliness of the teacher.

MORE JOAN RIVERS

My husband refused to participate in any way in the pregnancy . . . except the initial way. They thought of me as a divorcée in Lamaze class. I was looking forward to Edgar standing by my side, holding my hand, wiping my brow. Instead, he was standing at the vending machine, watching TV, or calling his mother. A complete zero in the delivery room! I never forgave him for that. My husband's dead 12 years and I'm still angry!

JOAN RIVERS

To ensure your graduation:

- **Don't plan on skipping many classes. They'll all hate you, including your wife, who must now explain your absence. They'll feel sorry for her and contempt for you. "What could he be doing that's more important? Why isn't he more supportive? Is that the best you could do for a husband?" My work took me out of town for 2 of the 12 classes, and I eagerly sought makeup dates with Gina and**

Mrs. Helfond. They communicated wordlessly in a way that sends the message that what's been missed can't possibly be made up and what you've lost will fall into the black hole of your knowledge forever. Hopefully, it won't come into play at birth time.

- Learn to help your wife with those special prenatal exercises like squatting and lying on her side. Do your best to keep a straight face while a roomful of pregnant women huff and puff their way through leg lifts.

- Help her with breathing techniques for labor. The commonly taught method is short, quick blowing motions in groups of three, followed by one long exhale: "ha, ha, ha, heeeeee." This will prove to be the most futile waste of time in the entire birth experience. When labor strikes for real, there will be much gasping and cursing. If there ever was a time a woman could be excused for bad language, surely childbirth is it. Birth class should include at least one lesson on Locker Room Potty-Mouth 101 because when it's time to deliver, your darling wife will have a vocabulary that would rot a hockey coach's tongue. She may go into labor a mild-mannered God-fearing girl from a nice family and quickly turn into a garbage-spewing cuss-meister whose language would have been censured at an

Osbourne Family Reunion. If you've never heard the "F-word" used as a noun, adverb, preposition, adjective, and dangling participle all in one sentence, eavesdrop on a delivery room one day.

- Investigate delivery options. You will hear about the many positions available, including (a) lying on your back with your knees in the air, (b) squatting and dropping the baby down vertically, (c) sitting in a bathtub at home, or (d) angling to your side and squeezing it out that way. (If your wife can pull this one off, she can tour next year with the Cirque du Soleil.)

  The deliveries are presented ultragraphically in a videotape shown at your third meeting. I made the mistake of attending that class fresh from work after stopping for take-out fried chicken. The aroma that made Colonel Sanders rich made me a pariah in a group of people watching placentas expunged ad nausea. By the time they got to the squatting video, I was squatting over Mrs. Helfond's commode. You will be discouraged from bringing food to birth class and will instead be offered carrot sticks, animal crackers, and the house wine, Gatorade. Be sure to order ahead.

- Cry on cue. After a few weeks the cumulative emotion of birth class is irresistible, and there won't be a dry seat in the house when they show tapes of the first moment of life. Just as I was getting all choked up, I smelled something burning in the garage, where Mrs. Helfond's kids had set fire to an old carpet.

- Learn the lingo. The language of birth represents great progress when you consider that our great grandmothers probably did not know what cervix meant . . . or effacement . . . or dilation. Do you? See how you fare by matching up the terms on the left with the multiple-choice meaning on the right.

1. downy lanugo
   a) a mudslide community in southern California
   b) the furry covering on the fetus's skin

2. waxy vernix
   a) a rapper from Jersey
   b) a vernix with wax on it
   c) a protective skinlike covering over the fetus while it is in the uterus

3. meconium
   a) semiprecious stones used in necklaces on the Home Shopping Network
   b) the tarlike waste that constitutes the newborn's first bowel movement

4. fetoscope light
    a) a new beer that tastes like baby pee
    b) a doctor's lamp that shines inside the uterus from which the baby will shield his eyes

5. amniotic waterbed
    a) where eels make love
    b) the bag of waters that surround and encase the fetus, a.k.a. amniotic sac

6. head-down position
    a) Tom Cruise in his car hiding from the parazzi the position you want for the baby as he's exiting the birth canal

7. group B streptococcus bacteria
    a) not as cool as group A but working on it a cousin of the bug that causes strep throat and can be fatal if passed to infants in the birth canal

8. immunoglobulin
    a) similar to supercalifragilistic a product of plasma cells that aids in fighting infection (If you're RH negative, get an RH immunoglobulin shot in the seventh month.)

MY WIFE, THE DOCTOR

Halfway through the course you think you are doing pretty well, but you are listening in awe to your wife's answers to Mrs. Helfond's quizzes and realizing that, comparatively speaking, she knows enough about childbirth to do her own infomerical. Where did she learn all this? It would take a crash course in obstetrics to keep up.

Here are some good questions to ask that'll make you look astute and curious.

- *What's the difference between breech, posterior, and anterior fetal positions?* In the breech fetal position, the baby emerges feet, knees, or buttocks first. This occurs in 3 percent of births. In the posterior fetal position, the baby is facing the wrong way, and the baby would be born face up. Anterior is the desired position during labor where the body is facing downward, toward the spine of the mother.

- *What causes fetal distress, and how do we handle it?* There is no way to know if the baby is in fetal distress if you are at home without a doctor. It is caused by a decrease in oxygen getting to the baby and can result from a cord wrapping around the baby's neck or from a malfunction in the placenta. Decreased fetal movement is usually, but not always, an indicator. It's like being in a room with the air-conditioning on: you're accustomed to the sound, so you don't notice it . . . until it shuts off and you

**become aware of the silence. Similarly, a
pregnant woman becomes accustomed to
activity from the baby, and if that suddenly
stopped, she would notice. Your wife can
monitor the baby by drinking eight ounces
of juice, lying down on her left side, and
counting fetal movements. Expect 6 to 10
movements in an hour; if no movement is
detected, call your doctor.**

"THIS IS ONLY A TEST . . . "

Your greatest concern is the one shared by every
other pregnant couple in the world, so let's get it on
the table now: 2 to 3 percent of newborns emerge with
a serious birth defect. Your nervousness can be
addressed by testing procedures such as the AFP
(alpha-fetoprotein) blood test, which will hopefully
eliminate any worries about open spinal defects or
Down syndrome. Discuss with your doctor which tests
you really need and why. Invasive procedures such as
chorionic villi sampling or amniocentesis carry a small
risk of miscarriage, and tests can have false positive
results that need to be interpreted by your obstetrician.
Most practitioners are confident with the results that
ultrasound monitoring offers—especially for younger
mothers—assessing fetal development and peeking in
on the placenta. Junior already has fingerprints, and by
now you may see your baby kick, roll, or even suck its

thumb. He or she is putting on some fat and has grown a coat of that waxy, whitish substance called vernix to protect the skin during residence in the amniotic fluid.

"I'M A PERSON, TOO!"

In month five, the fetus, now the size of a grapefruit, is tired of being a fish and a fruit and wants to be a person. The conscientious birth instructor wants you to begin relating to your baby as a real human being and will point out that he is starting to hear things in the womb, so mind your manners and watch your language. Loud noises can cause a muscle reflex in the fetus, whose heart rate may suddenly increase and whose limbs might flail around as if to say, "Can you change the channel or at least turn that down?" He will even hear Mom's stomach growling or her heart beating and will pick up a muffled version of her voice.

THE GRADUATING CLASS

Intentional or not, you are forming a bond with your birth classmates that will last a lifetime. You will always have something uniquely in common with these people, sharing as no one else does that brief window of time in which you all gave birth, thrust together with the singular thread being that all of your sperm and all of their eggs collided at the same time. Who knows? You may even have conceived during the same infomercial—that point in the tooth-whitening show where you get restless, and sex seems like an interesting alternative. Your young Michael or Jacob or Matthew will be born during the same week as their gorgeous Kaitlyn or Emily or Sarah. At first you are flush with excitement over the notion of bonding with your class-mates and will happily exchange numbers and plan reunions. I went so far as to propose a graduation prom, a cap and gown ceremony with me as valedictorian! They stared at me strangely and continued about their business.

"WHAT ARE YOU, A SNOB?"

You may soon conclude that the sperm collision theory is the only thing you have in common, however, when you all take a juice break and start talking about other subjects—like where you work or, worse yet, where he works. After 12 weeks, you may find your calendar so full that it will be impossible to find a night for the bunch of you to get together for a TV dinner at Skip and Wendy's trailer home.

Many classmates will want you to attend their baby's birthday party, and for the first year it's a lot of fun. The second year, there's a fishing derby on televi-sion. By the third year, you'd rather take a hot poker in the eyeball than force-feed one more platter of the macaroni and cheese Skip and Wendy's waif is now being raised on. Take a good look around the classroom and devise your social strategy before it's too late.

There will be at least one couple in class you really enjoy and identify with; one couple with the interests, humor, politics, and lifestyle you relate to. This will be the couple your wife hates most.

LAMAZE, BRADLEY, OR JACUZZI?

In 1853, Queen Victoria took chloroform for the birth of her eighth child, Prince Leopold, becoming the first woman to give birth under anesthetic. Her decision was against all religious doctrines and social customs of her time, but there followed an entire generation of women who opted to be knocked out, demanding twilight sleep to overcome pain and fear. A woman had become an unconscious object from whose pelvis a baby was extracted with no priority given to her feelings and emotions until the sixties, when women sought an active role in the birth of their babies.

In 1951, Dr. Fernand Lamaze introduced a method of childbirth in France by incorporating techniques he had observed in Russia. His classes emphasized the continuous emotional support of the husband and taught comfort measures such as hydrotherapy—the use of heat and cold and pressure—and relaxation skills, including breathing strategies that can be used throughout life in times of stress.

Women are taught how to focus and accept the pain of childbirth rather than fight it, making Dr. Lamaze one of the great public relations salesmen in history. For more information on Lamaze, get in touch with the American Society for Psychoprophylaxis in Obstetrics (ASPO/Lamaze) at its headquarters in Washington, DC. The Lamaze technique is taught in more than 150,000 classes annually in the United States, attended by approximately 2 million parents.

Another popular approach is the Bradley method. As a young obstetrician in the late 1940s, Robert Bradley was appalled by the heavy doses of medication commonly given during labor and believed that men should be integrated into the process as birth coaches— God love him! Today some 20,000 expectant couples enroll for Bradley instruction each year.

Bradley Dads are taught their own shorthand language as they encourage their laboring wives to "melt," "flow," "release," and "give in." Wives have been known to respond with their own ad-libs, including "shut up," "drop dead," "piss off," and "more drugs." It is the Bradley philosophy that teaches squatting as the most efficient way to give birth since it makes the best use of gravity and causes the least destruction of furniture.

BOOBOO LAMAZE

I had an intense 16-hour labor trying to deliver Cody without benefit of any painkillers because our anesthesiologist was enjoying himself at home with his own newborn. He figured my first delivery would take time, and he figured wrong. By the time he arrived I was 10 centimeters dilated and ready to push or, more accurately, ready to die. The only help I could hope for was from my Lamaze coach, the great world-class athlete, Frank Gifford. All he had to do—all he had to do—was count properly to monitor my breathing. Is that too much to ask? Apparently . . . because at one point during the agonizing process Frank lost his concentration and I lost my mind. I later forgave him when he went in for emergency back surgery, no doubt a result of bending over me for 16 hours.

KATHIE LEE GIFFORD, MOTHER OF CODY AND CASSIDY

*My Lamaze teacher had asthma—
she threw off our breathing!*

WIL SHRINER

NUTRITION

Birth class will emphasize the importance of a proper diet in the months to come, and, as husbands, we must support Mom's dietary regimen by at least eating her types of food, if not her quantities. A hint for the fellas is to not bother trying to keep up with the eating habits of a pregnant woman. It can't be done. Remember that she is eating for two, and if you try hanging with her, you will look like a Macy's Parade balloon. You might as well have "Goodyear" tattooed on your ass. A mother-to-be is capable of eating three balanced meals a day and 3-4,000 snacks in between.

The guidelines will represent a big adjustment for the macaroni and cheese crowd. Vegetarians will have an easier time adapting to a pregnancy menu because they are a more disciplined lot. Vegetarians don't care how food tastes, only "Did it pass easily?" Meat people like to savor food; vegetarians just want to get rid of it. "How was dinner?" "It felt good, and it's gone." That's a successful meal! "What did you have?" "I don't know; it felt like turnip." I compromised by becoming a semi-vegetarian . . . I eat only animals who eat vegetables.

Here is the ideal diet:

- **2,200 calories per day during the first three months**

- **2,500 calories per day during the second three months**

- **2,800 calories per day during the last three months**

General guidelines:

- **two or three servings daily of meat or other protein such as chicken, fish, peanut butter, or beans**

- **three or four servings daily of milk and other milk products**

- **four servings daily of fruits and vegetables**

- **four servings daily of whole-grain foods, such as rice, pasta, or whole-grain bread**

- **six to eight glasses of water, juice, or milk every day**

Baby boomers were taught to drink milk. We've since learned that dairy raises the cholesterol, so apparently my mom tried to kill me. Nevertheless, the calcium found in milk and dairy products does help build strong bones and teeth, prevents high blood pressure, promotes muscle contraction, and helps with blood clotting. Maybe the cow is our friend after all. Many vegetables contain calcium and can be substituted if dairy products prove difficult to digest.

MOTHERS!

- **Don't starve yourself. This is not the time to diet.**

- **Limit fatty, fried, and processed foods.**

- Limit foods and drinks with added sugar.

- Remember to avoid alcohol—some cold remedies contain alcohol—and avoid caffeine and ingesting too much of any one thing, including proteins and vitamins.

- Eat enough fish to accommodate your baby's brain development but not so much that you have to worry about mercury levels in the Great Lakes.

WORKING OUT

HER:
Help me exercise.

HIM:
I'll be glad to.

HER:
Are you saying I look fat?

HIM:
You look pregnant.

HER:
I told you we should have hired Rudy.

HIM:
*Mrs. Helfond said I could help you
get in condition for delivery.*

HER:
You usually just make fun of what she says.

HIM:
I'll go shingle the roof now.

There may come a time in the pregnancy of some couples at which the wife will weigh more than the husband. There is virtually no way for a man to make this observation without ending up with his head in the oven. Your wife may get such a jones for sugar and fat, you'll think she's on the Marlon Brando diet. Most women gain an average of 25 to 40 pounds, an amount that varies by 25 to 40 pounds. Of this, breast tissue may account for 10. (That extra 5 pounds per breast is one of the stats some women use to sell a man on pregnancy in the first place. She may go from beauty queen to Dairy Queen.)

Our wives can't look at their old bathing suits without becoming clinically depressed. Again, we can help by example. Maintain your own studlike demeanor, those throbbing pecs bursting through your alligator shirt like a thundering river in springtime. It may be helpful to know how many calories are burned in 30 minutes by a woman weighing 125 to 135 pounds.

Walking	**120 calories**
Bike riding	**180 calories**
Aerobic dancing	**180 calories**
Treadmilling	**300 calories**

You burn 150 calories making love and only 103 playing golf, unless you try a new position in a sand trap, in which case you can really do yourself some good. (You would think with the number of golf references in this book that I was good at it . . . I'm not. Golf is an exacting game, and I'm only an approximate guy. It takes a lot of balls to golf the way I do. My favorite part of the game is that you get to start a new hole every seven strokes.) Playing golf as a couple is a bad idea even when she's not pregnant because she probably hits too short, walks too slow, pees too much, and beats you!

ARE WE HAVING FUN YET?

Let's lighten the load and talk about the flip side, the part birth class understandably takes for granted. One of the reasons we have kids is that they're so darn much fun. The meaning of life becomes obvious, and the answer will soon appear before you: kids. Giving love is a beautiful thing, and being loved unconditionally in return is endlessly satisfying. The fact that someone trusts and depends on you so completely is a happy responsibility. Your child will make you feel strong, important, valuable, and tall. You will have an heir—someone who will carry on in your own stumbling manner and improve on it for another generation.

After slogging through the prenatal indoctrination, the money questions, the lifestyle considerations, you have earned the right to project into the future and reflect on some of the joy that lies ahead. Indulge yourself in the luxury of imagining your baby as he becomes your playmate, companion, and friend.

KIDS MAKE YOU LAUGH

General Rule: Other kids are annoying; yours are hilarious. When I took Brennan to the ballet for the first time—sure, like we attended regularly—he paid close attention as the girls danced around on their toes. When it was over, I asked, "How did you like it?" He said, "Fine, but why don't they just get taller girls?"

Robin once asked, "What does constipated mean?" I answered, "It means you can't go 'number 2.'" He said, "Why don't you just go number 1 twice?"

YOUR GROWING PAINS

Yes, you'll have them, as I had mine for seven years on TV. It would be cheating if I didn't take a few paragraphs to discuss my years on that show since it may be one of the reasons you bought this book. To refresh your memory, I played one of TV's favorite dads, based on an actual survey conducted among those members of my immediate family listed on the tax return as "dependents."

I am flattered that the two things everybody likes to talk to me about are *Growing Pains* and sex— *Growing Pains* because Leonardo DiCaprio was on it and sex because people just like to talk about it.

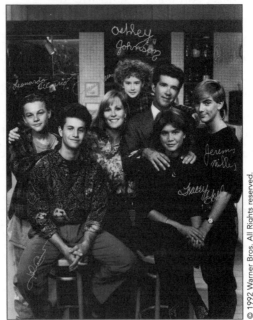

"Growing Pains," 1991

I was the one who told Leonardo, "Do a film about a boat with a problem!"

Dr. Jason Seaver was a psychiatrist whose advice to most patients was to go out and buy a nice sweater. As a parent, his solutions were more involved as he addressed situations that come up in most American families. My TV family was the best money can buy. When the show started in 1985, we had three children, which in California means one of each. Mike (Kirk Cameron) was a typical teenage boy, described as a hormone with feet. Kirk was more than a son to me; he was a residual. The show was a godsend, coming as it did on the heels of my first real-life divorce and affording me an opportunity to work in an environment that served as a playground for my real-life kids, who would visit after school and became friends with their same-age TV counterparts. Kirk and Tracey Gold and Jeremy Miller were fine role models for Brennan and Robin, and I wanted my kids to be just like them . . . rich!

My wife was played by a lovely actress named Joanna Kerns. (Remember "bookstore gas" in Month 2?) The tabloids speculated that we were having an off-screen affair, so for you inquiring minds who want to know, let me say that was not true. Joanna and I were not an item, we were not a romance, our relationship was purely sexual. (Sure, she wishes!) Joanna remains one of my dearest friends despite that remark. The reason the Seavers survived and triumphed in family management was simple: eight writers. Many parents feel intimidated by the families they see on television: wise, happy, sweet, effective, and humorous. Believe me, it's easy to make the right decisions with a committee of think-tankers putting words in your mouth. In real life, it's your kids who tell you how to parent.

Growing Pains was pretty realistic for the genre, but in a half-hour show the husband and wife must wake up in the morning and immediately start talking about the kids. This is before going to the bathroom. You never see a toilet on a sitcom. Either the Seavers had magic kidneys, or they were a very uptight family.

After talking about family problems, the Seavers kiss. This is before brushing their teeth, something you would never do to someone you planned on staying married to. In real life, I wake up feeling like Kobe Bryant left a sneaker in my mouth. Brushing and flushing are two emergencies that shouldn't be put off, and frankly there are times I'd rather tinkle than smooch.

On a sitcom, Dad's hair looks perfect. In real life, when I first sit up in bed, it's as if a Pomeranian exploded on my head. There are never any dead plants in a sitcom house. My house has no live ones. On TV, people have a problem, get a few laughs, kiss, and make up, all in 23 minutes. Come on . . . I've been married twice! In real life, you may not get a word in edgewise for two days.

On a sitcom, nobody ever locks the door or does any housework, and you make bigger faces than you'd make in real life. Try that wide-eyed deer-in-the-headlights look of astonishment in front of your kids, and they'll think you're a complete dork. On a sitcom, husband and wife look back and forth at one another knowingly. In real life, you look back and forth knowing nothing and hoping the other has a clue.

A sitcom can't tackle issues the same way the drama shows do, so you never see a smack on the head or a whack on the butt.

WHY IS THE BUNNY NOT BREATHING?

The only problem with Kirk Cameron as a role model was his boa constrictor. Children can learn about caring for all of God's creatures by having a pet in the house, but do yourself a favor and be involved in the selection of that pet.

Soon my son had to have a boa. I suggested to Kirk that he might get into pussycats or hamsters, and he did . . . but only as snake food. A boa's snack of choice is a mouse, which you bring from the pet store where he's been orpaned to what he thinks is his new home. He's thinking "cheese," and suddenly, zap, he's Mickey McMuffin. This can be shocking and disgusting, especially to the mouse, so if you consider a pet with a violent appetite, be sure your child understands that this activity is all part of nature's life cycle, or he'll be traumatized for life.

When she was four, my sister accidentally hugged our rabbit to death. Cuddled, smothered, and strangled him. The boa would have been proud.

HOW DO I KNOW HE'LL LOVE ME?

If you're wondering how long it will be before you start being scrutinized by yet another person in this world, count on your child to notice disturbing things about you at around six months. He will watch you entering and leaving a room, watch you hold an object and put it down. He is probably years away from overtly criticizing your every move, and it may be even longer before he actually expresses revulsion over everything you stand for, but later in your child's life he will find some of your mannerisms, voice tones, expressions, and even moods reflected in his own persona—things even bigger than drinking milk from the carton and cheating on his taxes. Approval from him will one day be the most important endorsement in your life, so plan to be a good person..

LEARN SOME SONGS

Kids intuitively love music, and it becomes an important communication tool as they respond to the various sounds in your voice. Be sure to brush up on the old standards like:

"I'm a Little Teapot"
"You Are My Sunshine"
"Twinkle, Twinkle Little Star"
"Row, Row, Row Your Boat"
"Doe, a Deer"

Feel free to use my new version of the alphabet song:

ABC, CNBC, VH-1, and BET
CBS, ESPN, PBS, and UPN
Now we've learned our MTV's
Let me watch the program, please!

I used to improvise songs for just about every occasion because the repetition seemed to help my boys learn the activity. "This is the way we wash our face," etc. Also, putting a musical happy face on a tumble or a scare always distracted them from the disaster part.

I taught my children how to laugh before I taught them words and duped them into thinking this was a legitimate form of expression. Consequently, their earliest sounds were not cries or whines but rather giggles and guffaws that filled our home with the sound of children's laughter. They paid me back later on by refusing to laugh at any of my jokes, complaining they were simply chuckled out.

WHEN DOES MAMA, DADA MEAN CACA?

One of the great moments in your life will be when your child first knowingly refers to you by name. In any language, a baby's first words usually feature the consonant b, p, or d because those sounds are the easiest to make. In the English language, you will likely hear

"Dada" or "Daddy"; in Spanish it's "Papa"; in Italian "Babo"; and the Chinese child will probably say "Ba."

It is your responsibility to interpret your baby to the outside world because you know him best and must tell others what he is thinking, saying, needing, wanting. When he says "Fata," does that mean "I'm hungry," "I'm thirsty," "I'm wet," "your breath stinks," "your hat is silly," or "get Uncle Festus's big hairy nose out of my face?"

A FATHER SMILES

> There's the smile you give your baby when you
>   hear that first sweet cry.
> Now explain that August birth; you just got
>   married in July.
> There's the smile of pride when all the school-
>   boys want to date your daughter.
> Just don't let you find their fingerprints on that
>   new dress you bought her.
> Your son is in his first parade, he smiles from ear
>   to ear,
> Bends down to tie his shoes, and gets a
>   trumpet up the rear.
> You smiled at his first touchdown though his
>   clothes were such a mess.
> What you don't know is underneath he wears
>   his sister's dress.
> You'll smile for every tear, for all the good times
>   and the bad,

But nothing beats the time he says, "I want to be like Dad."

FACTS

- Chlorine can be harmful to a developing fetus.

- Pregnant women should not only shower off after taking a swim but before taking the plunge as well because new research indicates that chlorine can be even more dangerous when mixing with skin care products.

- In 1901, Queen Victoria died, but not before counseling women on how to endure the act of sex: "Lie back and think of England."

- Porcupines are born with quills—a terrifying concept—but they're soft and only harden with age.

- The gestation period for a duck-billed-platypus is 10 days. Irrelevant, but I knew you'd be envious.

- The average American woman is 5'4' and weighs 142 pounds. The average model is 5'9" and weighs 110 pounds.

- In her eighth month, Gina went out to the swimming pool, got on a float and sank it. 'Nuff said.

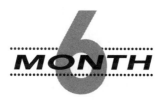

MONTH 6

FEAR

The sixth month is a good time for a glucose screen that would detect gestational diabetes—a temporary condition that can be controlled by diet and exercise and will subside within two weeks after you give birth. Mother-to-be may feel baby-to-be having hiccups—a perfectly natural occurrence and a reminder of how completely integrated her life is with that of your unborn child.

"I WANT TO TALK TO MY KID!"

At the next ultrasound, you will see fingers moving, legs kicking, and the heart beating. Most significantly, you may now *determine the sex if you want to!* Again, make sure a professional is helping you interpret these images, because what looks like a penis could actually be a finger. If, when he grows up, his finger still looks like a penis, teach him not to point.

Having lost the "let's find out" battle, I was at least determined not to get this momentous news in the sterile environment of an OB/GYN's examining room. Rather, we instructed the doctor to type in the sex on the ultrasound videotape so we could play it at our chosen time. That time was the next weekend at a fundraiser in Colorado with President Gerald Ford. We played the tape before dinner. Then I got bold enough at the banquet to approach him and ask for an autograph to "Carter,"(for Carter would be his name) and "To Carter from Ford" would be a presidential classic as a first autograph.

The baby-to-be is now approximately 30 centimeters long and will continue to grow by approximately 5 centimeters monthly. Your baby weighs 1 pound, whereas you and your wife have each gained 20. At this rate, if he weighs 8 pounds, you'll gain 160. Don't worry; that's not how it works. This 20-to-1 ratio, however, is a good measuring stick for what it takes to raise a child. Like traveling with 20 baby bags for every one of yours—car seats, strollers, food, and diaper containers. Plan to leave the nanny behind and hire a Sherpa. She may even pack suitcases filled with your child's blankets, pillows, and toys so that during your vacation he'll have continuity. You'll point out that's what parents are for. She'll point to your old pal, the sofa, if you want a good night's sleep.

Back on the subject of weight gain, if she's pushing the envelope, your doctor will want you to slow her down this month. If it was difficult to discuss earlier, it's suicidal now. She may say she's pleased with her weight. Fat people say they like being that way in case they crash-land in the Peruvian Alps and have to eat one of their toes. Your wife has no such excuse.

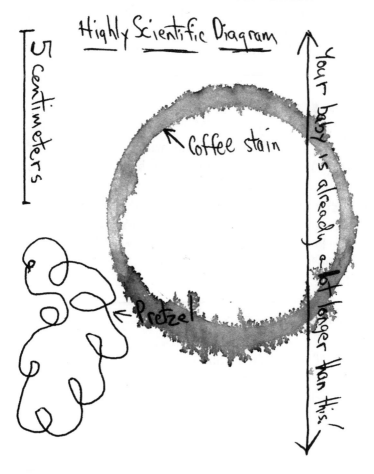

Highly Scientific Diagram

5 centimeters

← Coffee stain

← Pretzel

Your baby is already a lot longer than this!

Maybe she'll get the hint herself if her sweatpants start sweating before she gets into them . . . if she goes bicycling and her cheeks get caught in the spokes . . . she'll catch on.

Remember the possible connection between excessive weight gain, baby weight, and diabetes? Being too heavy can also cause hypertension, fetal growth retardation, placental insufficiency, and surgical complications due to mal-presentation (i.e., the baby in breech or anterior position).

"I'M SCARED!"

Of course you are. Your wife is going to have a baby! You are more pumped up than you've ever been about anything in your life. (Not a Viagra joke.) In three months, you'll have a son or daughter, and as the excitement mounts, so does the anxiety. Stop worrying. People dumber than you have been doing this for centuries.

"SHE'S SCARED!"

Of course she is. She's afraid you might flake, fold, flip, flop, or faint. She may have other concerns you can help with.

- *Fear that her water will break in public.* This may be her best chance ever to get back at you for all those obnoxious bodily functions you claim are unavoidable. History shows that men enjoy belching, and to many this constitutes their entire sense of humor. Although some men belch randomly in front of total strangers, others burp more selectively in front of nieces and nephews, preferring to perform at family gatherings where the wife can be humiliated in front of her relatives. Timing her water to break at a dinner meeting with her husband's boss could even the score for years of offensive Thanksgivings and ensure a family anecdote for generations to come. Regrettably for her sake, only one in seven women's membranes ruptures before the onset of labor. Rest assured, if it happens while you're out and about, she will have the highly identifiable "My bag of waters just broke" look on her face, and no one will mistake this development for incontinence.

- *Fear you won't know when you're in labor.* It is also possible that you would not recognize when a tornado rips the roof off your house and tosses a cow in your backyard, when you lose your leg in a grizzly bear attack, or . . . your prostate examination. Barring a frontal lobotomy earlier that day, a woman will likely know when she's in labor.

If you wanted a hospital birth and it's a false alarm, the worst that could happen is you'll show up and then be sent home for a while.

- *Fear of behaving badly during childbirth.* We've discussed colorful language, but your wife may now be concerned about soiling the bed or slugging her mate. How 'bout soiling the whole room and slugging the nurse, the doctor, the husband, and some innocent passersby? It's all possible in the wild and wacky world of labor, but don't worry: in the heat of battle, she won't care, and you can be sure your medical team has seen it all.

- *Fear of stretch marks.* Be flattered that this trepidation is really about you. She wants to continue being beautiful for her husband and is afraid she will be less Gwyneth Paltrow–like if her future body harbors those unmistakable battle scars of childbirth. Keep in mind that her concern about your reaction to stretch marks is well founded in your long history of shallowness. If all you seem to care about is sex, shape, weight, skin tone, and the Hawaiian Tropic Pageant on Pay Per View, she has good reason to expect your callousness at the postpartum sight of . . . you-know-what. (You can practice political correctness by referring to them as laterally enhanced epidermal elasticity residuals.) Assure her that although most women get them, many epidermal separations fade in time to a much lighter beige line. Deep down inside, you will find these badges of honor to be a reminder of the fabulous child you've been blessed with and the woman who gave you this gift, more of a woman now than she's ever been, and because of her, you are more of a man.

• *Fear that she will lose her vaginal muscles.* This one always gets the guys' attention. Unless you're planning a penile enlargement, it is possible that you could notice a discrepancy in your postpartum "fit." It will be reassuring for both of you to remember that a small incision and a few stitches applied shortly after delivery can restore the original size of the beloved aperture. For a "natural" approach, Kegel exercises will help strengthen pelvic muscles, assisting both delivery and postpartum recovery. Dr. Kegel later discovered that his exercises increased orgasm intensity. It is for his work in this field that the kindly doctor should be regarded by grateful couples in the same reverent light as Louis Pasteur, Madame Curie, and Dr. Christiaan Barnard. No doubt the time will come when Kegel cultists will have a holiday declared in their hero's name,

meeting perhaps at a ball game for a
commemorative hot dog in a symbolically
snug bun.

FEAR OF PARENTING

The Big One. Afterbirth is more than a mess; it's a
way of life! On modifying your lifestyle. . . .

- *At what temperature should we maintain
  our household?* Answer: 72 degrees should
  be comfortable for the whole family. If an
  infant's hands or feet seem cold, it's because
  the vascular system will not be fully developed until after the third month of life. A
  cold is caused by a virus, and there is no evidence that a cooler temperature makes the
  baby more susceptible to illness. It's all
  about germs, germs, germs. If your newborn is fussy and can't be comforted by
  feeding or cuddling, that's a more reliable
  indication that it's too warm or cold.

- *Should the newborn sleep in his own room?*
  This is a matter of personal preference as
  long as the baby has a firm mattress and is
  put down on his back to avoid SIDS.

On cribs, the bars should be no more than 2⅜ inches apart to prevent a baby's head from getting stuck in between. The mattress should fit snugly so the head can't slide down between the mattress and the side of the crib. All surfaces should be smooth, and the railing should be two feet higher than the mattress, unless of course the baby is three feet tall at birth, in which case get him a higher railing and a basketball. (Your child-proofer should have caught these points, but it's your baby, so check once, check twice, then check again.) A foam mattress is recommended by many pediatricians in case the baby has allergies to other stuffings.

- *What loud noises should I worry about?* If a jet engine were to start up in the room next to the nursery, you would have something to be concerned about. Otherwise, ordinary household sounds such as the vacuum cleaner, radio, TV, or dog barking pose no risk of hearing damage.

- *Should our baby be protected from visitors and their germs?* Known lepers should be discouraged from casually dropping by. Neighbors or relatives with symptoms of infection such as a runny nose or fever should also be kept away. Otherwise, simple handwashing will take care of most exposure problems, and new parents can take comfort in the fact that newborns are not as

> fragile as you'd expect and will be develop-
> ing their own immune system in the early
> months. This is especially true of a breast-
> fed infant, who has the additional antibodies
> he's getting from Mom.

- *Should we feed the baby by breast or bottle?*
  Breast-feeding is always handier for a
  woman, and even the most ambitious husbands should stick with the bottle method.

Babies are born with a rooting reflex and will turn
in the direction of a touch to the cheek. When to feed
will be no mystery because a hungry baby will turn
toward the nipple with an open mouth. This instinct
will subside around the time of (a) six months, (b) two
years, or (c) college graduation.

GOT MILK?

> Every night at about 4:00 a.m. I would be attempt-
> ing to breast-feed Cody when, for some reason, he
> would refuse to nurse from my left breast (everyone's a
> critic). If there is anything more painful than an engorged
> breast, I hope it never happens to anyone I love! It's
> massive and it's menacing, and it seemed the only
> means of relief would be a breast pump. Good idea,
> except . . . the sound of Frank's snoring in rhythm with
> the sucking sound of that wretched breast pump was
> the postnatal equivalent of Chinese water torture.
>
> KATHIE LEE GIFFORD

- *What other reflexes should I look for?* A healthy baby will exhibit reflex grasping, grabbing your finger and holding on tight. Via reflex head control, infants lying face down can lift and turn their heads to breathe, a nifty survival skill. In the Morrow reflex, infants react to sudden physical sensations and loud noises by throwing their arms and legs up as if to signal touchdown. Reflex walking takes place when you hold your infant with his feet touching a surface. Your baby will take a few steps even though he won't have the strength to support himself for about a year.

Other instinctive reflexes include:

a. the ability to know exactly when you're finally nodding off to sleep so they can begin howling

b. knowing that when the diaper comes off and the cold air hits is a perfect time to pull the trigger on the squirt gun

c. Reflex burping—as soon as you put on a clean shirt

- *What do I do when my baby won't stop crying?* One of the following does not belong: (a) soothing him in a rocking chair, (b) putting your baby across your knees and rubbing his back, (c) taking a stroll with the baby carriage, (d) going for a ride in the car, (e) winding up the music box mobile hanging over the crib, (f) offering a pacifier, (g) drinking a fifth of bourbon. There are different kinds of cries: the cry of hunger, the cry of illness or pain, the cry of shock, a fussy teething cry, a midnight can't-sleep cry, and a manipulative whine.

- *What can my newborn baby see?* Colors, shapes, patterns, movement, and light. They are nearsighted and prefer objects 8 to 12 inches from their faces.

- *When do I trim his nails?* While he's sleeping soundly.

- *Does iron cause constipation?* There is no firm evidence of this, but it's a good idea not to let your child eat a shovel since it is difficult to pass, even though it might come in handy cleaning up the mess.

- *Does thumb sucking result in buck teeth?* Thumb sucking is usually okay as long as it's the baby's own thumb and he stops by around age five. Sixteen-year-olds sucking the thumbs of total strangers is frowned on and could lead to intervention by a security guard. Your pediatrician will explain that infant thumb sucking is a common, normal way of courting the sucking reflex.

- *Do babies who walk early become bow-legged?* Nope. Babies who walk early are simply walking early.

- *Will a fat baby be a fat grown-up?* Not necessarily. Babies need a lot of baby fat, and a fat baby will become a fat adult only if his fat parents keep feeding him fat foods throughout his fat life, so set a big fat example by your own eating habits, but don't worry about the kid for the first few years.

- *What can we do to help intelligence develop?* (a) Have a smarter person move in, (b) provide a stimulating environment, and (c) play age-appropriate games.

- *What do I do in the event of an emergency?* That depends on the emergency, but never throw a drowning person a sponge. An educated parent is a calm and effective one. An unenlightened parent will tend to panic six to eight times daily, call the pediatrician twice a week, and dial 911 before the kid's a month old. This can be a drain on Mom and Dad and a nuisance to medical personnel in your area.

The more you know, the more you can analyze and diagnose and the more qualified you'll be to recognize real problems when they arise. See if you can recognize true emergencies from fake ones among the following.

a.   Your child has a cough. A true emergency.
     True or false? (false)

b.   Your child has a rash. A true emergency.
     True or false? (false)

c.   On your visit to Australia, you can't find
     your toddler, and a pack of dingoes is
     circling the tent. (Call 911.)

d.   Your Toyota is heading down the driveway
     with your three-year-old at the wheel, and
     you know for a fact he doesn't have a
     license. (Double the panic if it's leased.)

e.   Your child has a startled look on his face,
     and his hair is in flames. (Duh!)

•   *My six-month-old makes coughing sounds,
    but I know very well he's not sick. Why is he
    faking that?* Your child is a liar and a fraud
    and will have a great career in politics or
    telemarketing. Or . . . your baby is enter-
    taining himself and realizing that he assumes
    an element of control by making a new
    sound that you respond to. He is experi-
    menting with his own body and learning
    how to get reactions out of the world
    around him.

•   *My nine-month-old babbles when she wakes
    up in the morning.* We are delighted that
    she no longer cries, but why the babbling?

**Clearly, your child is delusional and has no
grip on reality. She will have a fine career
as an actress or stock analyst. Or . . . the
baby's highest intellectual level is in early
morning when she first wakes up, and this
babbling is another example of playing with
sound capabilities—and you'd know this if
you were paying attention three months ago
during that coughing experiment.**

TALK TO ME ABOUT SLIMY BLACK MOLD

One cause of chronic sniffling and respiratory difficulty can be the kind of household mold that flourishes
unseen in damp areas. Most couples are likely to notice
things like a flood or a dead body in their basement, but
minor water damage can cause mold under carpets, in air
conditioners, or within walls or ceilings, and the mold
releases spores into the air, which can irritate and inflame.
Children with asthma and allergies are especially vulnerable, and if the slimy black mold is more than you can clean
up with bleach and water and blow dryers, consult the
Health Department or a professional contractor. (I have
no good references for the latter.)

WHEN TO SAY "NO"

When my youngest passed the six-month mile-stone, he began passing a lot of other things, too. A six-month-old is a vessel, a container. You pour things in until he overflows, which is his way of saying, "I'm full," then he leaks, dribbles, spits, or sometimes explodes in cataclysmic eruptions of thermonuclear proportions. His body is ingesting different foods and more of them, so when a six-month-old has a bowel movement that hits 4.2 on the Richter scale, you learn to run and stand in the doorway.

The major psychological change at this age is that he's about to hear the word "no" for the first time. If you put yourself in his booties, surely this is the most traumatic and defining event in life. Until now, he has been encouraged to do whatever he pleases without limitation. "Come on, make a noise. Let's see you use your hand. Grab this, hold that, the world is yours, and so is everything in it."

Suddenly when he can actually make a loud sound or touch something breakable, he hears the word no.

KID:

Hey, wait a minute! Yesterday I squeezed your finger and I was a hero; you were bringing friends by, and I was getting applause. Now I push a vase off the coffee table, and I'm a schmuck. Were you just kidding? I've been lied to, suckered, duped! Damn!

It's the End of the Innocence.

DON HENLEY

WHEN THEY SAY "OUCH!"

A parent's most helpless feeling is when your child is in pain; it starts with colic or teething and builds from there. Ideas for alleviating your child's pain include empathy, comfort, distraction, imagination, and fantasy.

I mentioned Brennan being diagnosed with diabetes at the age of four, and after enduring about a month of blood testing and insulin injections, he had simply had enough. He cried and I cajoled. He kicked me away and I kept checking my watch, knowing he needed a shot to balance his blood sugar. After two hours of tenderness, toughness, reasoning, wrestling, and begging, I finally had to pin him down and give him the needle. His tortured wail cut to the bottom of my heart. He couldn't know that my forcefulness was for his own good, and I too began to cry. When Brennan saw my pain, his attitude changed. He softened and concluded that Daddy meant no harm, that this process was tough on both of us. The tears stopped, and he held out his arms and hugged me as if to say, "I guess we're in this together, Dad." From that point on, the needles still hurt, but our hearts were healed and he had a friend with whom to share that suffering twice a day.

FEAR YOU'LL BE MISTAKEN
FOR THE GRANDFATHER

There seem to be fewer rules these days about the ages at which men, and for that matter women, can have babies. A 61-year-old woman gave birth this decade, although why anyone that old would want to do so remains a mystery. Shouldn't she be playing bridge on a cruise ship and checking out nursing homes instead of preschools? Apparently not. More kids is an easier concept for men because they don't have the pain of childbirth and by age 50 have probably recovered from the pain of divorce and the pain from a previous set of children breaking your heart by either siding with the mother, hounding you for more cash, or marrying unsuccessfully themselves, thus repeating the cycle and proving that marital failure might be genetic.

So why not do it again? No good reason. Just be sure if you're considering joining the Fathers at 50 Club that you think ahead to the day when you'll be sitting on the porch with a blanket over your legs, watching Junior play baseball while you try to stay awake for 10 minutes at a time, which is as long as you can do anything anymore. In fact, the reason you call him "Junior" is because you can place the face but occasionally not his name. As the nurse wipes oatmeal off your chin and blows your nose, you'll want to be secure in the knowledge that your insurance is paid up and your late-in-life offspring will be taken care of, whatever his name is.

"I THINK WE SHOULD START SEEING OTHER PEOPLE"

No. Don't turn your back now! It's possible that both of you are having nightmares reflecting your total lack of fitness to be parents. My wife dreamed that she forgot to feed the baby and he shriveled up like a spent balloon. Coincidentally, I had a reverse balloon dream that I had overfed him until he puffed up and exploded, flying around the room and finally coming to rest like a puddle with eyes. It never happened. Relax. It's getting closer, and you are so caught up in the excitement that your priorities are starting to change. Your work no longer dominates your every thought, you're not thinking as much about your boat, and you don't care that the Knicks blew another close one or that Washington is passing bills without your approval. More and more, your world is narrowing in a beautiful way to focus on your wife and baby and all the loving feelings they are stirring in you.

Panel

*Her most outrageous behavior during labor
was hollering directions.
She had one friend shooting stills,
another with a video camera,
and me working a tape recorder.
She was setting up the shots
and telling the doctor where to stand.
I had to remind her
she was also having the babies.*

Bob Seagren

Facts

- At age 40, half of a woman's eggs are chromosomally abnormal, at 42, that figure is 90 percent.

- Once a woman celebrates her 42nd birthday the chances of her having a baby using her own eggs is less than 10 percent.

- Only one in a thousand babies in the U.S. is born to a woman age 45 or over.

- 1 in 5 women between the ages of 40 and 44 is childless.

- Fifty-three percent of full-time working boomer mothers say they're too busy to have fun, compared to 36 percent of boomer fathers.

- Births happen most commonly in the United States on Tuesdays (average 12,000 a day); least commonly on Sundays (average 8,000).

- Infants cannot shed tears until they are three months old.

- Disposable diapers were invented in 1946.

- Wearing vertical stripes to hide girth only makes you look like a tall fat person.

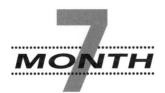

MONTH

SEX

Finally! If you've skipped ahead and started at this month, you've missed a lot of helpful tips, so go back.

Sex during pregnancy will not be a problem unless the husband wants to have some. Sex won't be a *big* problem unless the husband really likes it a lot. The truth is, most healthy women can continue to have sexual intercourse throughout their pregnancy, and if we all work together—doctors, counselors, husbands, and friends—maybe we can convince them of this. Of the many sacrifices that come with having a child, at the top of the list is sex.

It will come as no surprise that diminished or compromised sexual activity will be more of a problem for guys than women. Already in the first six months, you have no doubt experienced some major differences, such as her libido not quite keeping up to yours, the old positions you can't do because of the belly factor, and the new techniques you've had to master to make anything happen. The big advice in this seventh month is "Get it now! Last usable organ for one hundred miles." Enjoy what you can while you can because the shop may be closing down until further notice.

If there is one theme you are picking up on in your reading, it is that there are no certainties, no rules, no guarantees, patterns, or formulas outlining pregnant-hood. It is a very personal experience and different for every couple.

In no aspect is the variable more pronounced than in sex. There are grand differences from woman to woman and even for the same woman from day to day, month to month, pregnancy to pregnancy. If you con-centrate, there may be some lessons learned during this period that could improve your sex life even after the baby is born. Pregnancy may be the first time in a man's life when he's had to be truly unselfish, thought-ful, understanding, or caring to get laid, instead of just pretending to be.

FACTS

- It's not that men like sex more, but we do like more sex.

- It is tougher being the host organ than the donor organ.

Back in the second and third months, morning sickness probably killed much of her sex drive. That was okay for you because, as kinky as you are, not many guys get hot over getting barfed on. Even when she's feeling better, some couples might be nervous about indulging if they've had any difficulty conceiving or have experienced a miscarriage, in which case the doctor might advise temporary abstinence. Restraint may also be in order if your wife experiences vaginal bleeding, if either of you has had a sexually transmitted disease, or if you are expecting twins or triplets.

Can sex trigger labor? It is true that stimulation can promote the release of a hormone that causes contractions late in the pregnancy, but remember, contractions are not necessarily synonymous with labor. One theory you might want to promote is that pregnant women experience stronger orgasms because of increased blood flow to the friendly regions.

Does oral sex during pregnancy pose a problem? The answer is a resounding no. Cunnilingus is not a threat as long as you don't blow air into the vagina. This would seem a curious practice regardless, but certainly pregnancy is no time to pretend that your wife is a trombone. Be gentle.

As a father-to-be, you may have your own sexual concerns, such as wondering if you should hold back for fear of harming the fetus. How would you like to be him, look out your door, and see one of those things coming at you? Don't flatter yourself. The baby is safely tucked away in a manner that God invented to

protect this little angel, even from the imposing mag-
nitude of your surging manliness.

You may have difficulty relating to the new image
of your sex goddess when she hits her earth-mother
stride full on. This transition may cause some confusion
in your own sexual response, but get over it. Like the
(pardon the expression) stretch mark adjustment, you
will feel more mature if you experience fetal attraction—
that sensation of genuinely finding the expectant mom
look to be sexy. For the future, a woman who can be both
vamp and earth mother can be a deeper, richer, even
more exciting package for the well-rounded male.

THE SUPERWOMAN CATEGORY

Then there is the woman who finds her libido on
fire due to the raging hormones now affecting her
breasts, vagina, labia, and clitoris, heightening her
sensitivity and sexual readiness. The women overcome
with this phenomenon, positively touched by the
fertility muse and under the spell of the goddess of
excitation, will feel hornier than they've ever been,
masturbating frequently, wanting to be serviced several times a day, and experiencing multiple orgasms. This
woman is married to the guy next door. Your wife is in
the "touch me and die" category. Those are the breaks.

She may sense you're feeling neglected, unloved,
unattractive, and all those other little boy things that
have always worked when you sulked to get your way.

Those tricks just don't cut it anymore, however, because she has a larger agenda, there's no time to play games, and her needs must come first. Encourage your wife to talk about her sexual feelings even if they are negative or indifferent. Remember, it's just a phase she's going through that could be over in 15 to 18 years!

Your wife will remind you that there are other ways to express affection and to be intimate without having intercourse. Women assure us that touching, massaging, and cuddling can take the place of *hammertime*. Clearly, women don't get it, and this will forever be one of those areas in which men are from Mars and women don't dig Martians. A guy knows there is no substitute for the real thing, no mock nookie, no faux boffing. Nevertheless, for now let it be her call.

MEN REALLY WANT TO BE SUPPORTIVE, SYMPATHETIC, UNDERSTANDING, AND PATIENT. HONEST!

HE:
I understand you're in pain, sweetheart . . . so when?

SHE:
I'd love to, baby. It's just that I feel so bloated these days.

HE:

I know, sweetheart. It must be uncomfortable . . . so when?

SHE:

I just don't think I could concentrate. There's so much on my mind.

HE:

Of course you're distracted . . . so when?

SHE:

The timing's not right, you know? Our sex has always been so special, and I wouldn't want it to become a thing where I actually get turned off. I mean, I know you don't do it on purpose, but well . . . uh . . . I'm feeling a little pressured and . . . I'm turned off! I'm really turned off, so don't bug me!

HE:

I hear ya. You're turned off. So when?

Start thinking about the next six months as a month called "Mr. Happy Hibernates." It would be best to put your own libido into a deep sleep and focus on those more spiritual elements of your relationship.

If you have any sex in the eighth and ninth months, it's probably because she considers you a charity case, a forlorn waif left alone on the highway of love who needs emergency roadside service from a Good Samaritan wearing that perfume you adore.

Having said that, you may still have a shot at a couple of mid- to late-pregnancy pops if you play your cards right. If intercourse is the goal (and when is it not?), it may require some acrobatic, athletic improvisation in your positioning such as the side-by-side approach or the woman on top or on her knees with the man **behind.** I don't want to get too graphic here; suffice it to say that you may want to invest in a forklift, a trampoline, a circus swing, a rope and pulley apparatus, and a net. And learn some special stretching exercises from your chiropractor.

> *It was like mating with Shamu.*
>
> WIL SHRINER

"SO WHEN?"

Your doctor will likely tell you that intercourse is possible as early as six weeks after delivery. Upon hearing this, your wife may want to switch doctors. This is not the kind of scientific support she was counting on. For six weeks after childbirth, she'll have the substantial excuses of risking uterine infection or damaging the episiotomy stitches or general uncertainty if there is still any bleeding.

In truth, she is simply not of a mind to feel romantic for at least a couple of months. Her hormone levels have dropped like a bad day on the Nasdaq, causing the vaginal lining to dehydrate. If she is breast-feeding, the increase in milk production results in lower levels of estrogen. Where is that pesky hormone when you need it?

Estrogen's positive contribution is in its role as lubricator, although you can expect to require some extra help in the form of water-soluble gels or lubricated condoms when you do start your engines again. A little extra time in foreplay would also be a nice idea to give all of her responses a chance to kick in. If extra foreplay for you means expanding your two-minute drill, you probably need rehabilitative coaching anyway, and a refresher course will come in handy.

A BAD IDEA

In Ghana, it is taboo to have intercourse during pregnancy and for at least two years after birth. This is to ensure that the mother does not pick another seed before the child is old enough to be weaned. It is their approach to family planning.

A GOOD IDEA

This is why their society is polygamous, to avoid the strain that the man would certainly go through during this long period of abstinence.

ADAM VERSUS EVE

JOKE:
*What type of food causes a woman
to lose her sex drive?*

Wedding cake!

At the precise time you are selfishly singing, "I can't get no . . . satisfaction," she may be going through an intensely spiritual phase inspired by her role in the pro-creation of the species.

As touched as you are by her spirituality—it is one of the qualities that made you fall in love in the first place—you will nevertheless want to come back to "So when?" If, when nature takes its course, the course doesn't begin with inter, one last resort could be the transparently self-serving chestnut:

"Honey, making love will distract you from your discomfort." Don't be surprised if she chooses shopping instead.

THE DEFINITION OF CELIBACY

Celibate means "cranky." It will be necessary, how-ever, and you must practice this art with grace and good humor. If there is one aspect of his pregnancy you ladies might try to empathize with, understanding those frustrated sexual feelings will be among the most important. His sexuality is, after all, where he hides his ego and his self-worth and validation about his attractiveness and his intelligence. What it comes down to is "If you don't want me now, this minute, hot and nasty, then I guess I'm not very lovable." Remember this simple-minded thinking is not done by the head that wears a hat. Take it as a grand compliment that he desires you so and misses your carnal companionship.

ATTENTION, MOTHERS!

Understanding your husband's sexuality will help in the event you have a male child whose adolescence will become your problem in 13 years.

> **If your kids don't run away**
> **from home during puberty,**
> **you should.**
> **There is no known cure.**
>
> GOD

I tried explaining sex to Robin when he was 11, and he nodded his head, seeming to get it, until I asked if he had any questions. "Yes," he said. "Why would anyone want to do that?" I explained further, asked again, and this time got "Okay, Dad, but how do you keep from laughing?" I figured he was still a couple of years away.

When Brennan was 13, I wasn't worried about his having sex because his room was too messy. There was no place to lie down. It looked like the last days of Pompeii. Crows would dive under the bed looking for edible fungus and find it.

The one hope you have in delaying a young man's obsession with sex is his preoccupation with flatulence. If your sons are more interested in gas than girls, you are safe. Gas keeps boys away from girls—and vice versa. Young boys become absolutely giddy at the thought of passing wind. They have contests—the bigger, the louder, the nastier the explosion, the better. If you blow an O-ring, you're in the *Blazing Saddles* Hall of Fame. Encourage gas, folks; the smell is a small price to pay for your peace of mind.

When your boy stops tooting and starts putting away his crusty socks, it's time to hose him down, Scotchgard his underwear, and put speed bumps on his braces. Nothing helps. When teenage boys go upstairs and lock the door, you hope they're cutting cheese, or you can bet the time has come. The magazines suddenly appear from under the bed, steam flows from around the door, the walls begin throbbing, and you'll soon have to call the paramedics to come pump a Britney Spears poster out of some kid's stomach.

When a boy turns 14, he is a human sexual time bomb, ready to go off at any moment. His shorts come with a warning label, and his pants come into the room 10 seconds before he does. For the rest of his life, those pants will tell him what to do, where to go, how to spend his money. You try talking to him, but he's listening to his pants, so save your breath, because *his pants have a mind of their own* (another good country song).

Sudden changes in fashion—like the Franco-Prussian look—can be a warning sign that the dreaded "P-word" is on the horizon. When he puts so much mousse in his hair that caribou follow him home, coming of age is coming to your house. It is a known fact that a 15-year-old boy can jump-start a car with his tongue, and if his new career goal is to be the official gynecologist for the next Olympics, he's ready to go skinny-dipping in the gene pool.

SEX AND GOVERNMENT

Congress is constantly proposing new legislation for meat inspection, traffic offenses, immigration, and school prayer. What parents need is a law that says you must get a license to have sex. A beginner's permit. Help! Take the responsibility out of your hands when your son says, "Michael's parents let him lock the door when his girlfriend is in the room." "Hey, Mom and I would love for you and Tammy to spend the night, but sorry, it's the law."

The legal driving age is 16. You can say, "I'd let you get behind the wheel, but the mean ol' State of California won't. If it were me, you woulda been driving when you were four—it's those darn elected officials."

You can't drink until you're 18 or 21, so when he

says to you at 17, "Dad, it's just a couple of beers," you can say, "I know you're a man, I wanted to see you drunk as a skunk at the age of 9, but those old fogey legislators . . . no can do!"

Military service? Gotta be 18.

How did they get all these laws on the books and miss the big one? Let's campaign for a minimum age for sex! And what should that age be? I think 75. And then you can do it only if there's a parent in the room. We'll be 110 and won't remember the problem!

ADVISORY

Girls tend to think boys are out for only one thing. They are wrong. Boys are out for everything. When a boy sees a beautiful girl in zip-lock pants with bosoms that babies cry for, looking so good that when she sits down the chair smiles, his ego will make promises the rest of him can't keep. "I'll light your fire, rock your world, float your boat." This is usually a case of premature exaggeration.

For males, the mystery of sex is simple: "Who can I do it with?" "Yes or no?"—that's the mystery. Books tell us how to, why to, what to, when to, where to. What boys really want to know is "who to?" Kids must be careful about sexual disease in an era when a simple cold sore seems like the good old days. When a girl says she's going to give you something to remember her by, you better hope it's a nice tie (presidents excepted).

BOY QUIZ

When my son has his first non-urinary-related erection, I will:

a) **explain what is happening**

b) **measure it**

c) **have a parade**

d) **see if he knows what caused it and hope it's not the neighbor's Rottweiler**

GIRL QUIZ

Having chauvinistically referred to your baby as "him" throughout, let me switch genders and offer this test on the subject of raising girls, about which I have no direct knowledge.

When my daughter has her first period, I will:

a) **make sure she understands what's happening and is pleased with it**

b) **lock her in her room for the rest of her life**

c) **slaughter a goat and say a prayer**

When my daughter brings home her first date, I will:

a) **welcome him into our home and congratulate his good taste**

b) slip him a condom

c) kill the bastard

"Does she have to be a teenager?"

If you have a daughter, someday, yes. Dear Parents of Girls: Don't think your daughter has been a good girl just because she comes home from a date with a Gideon Bible in her purse.

BOYS WILL BE BOYS, AND THAT CAN GET YOU PREGNANT

In defense of boys, it still takes two to tangle, and outside California that second person will often be a girl.

Statistics tell us that in the year 2010 a teenage girl will get pregnant every 35 seconds. This girl must be stopped!

When a man finally meets the perfect lover, you gotta ask, "How did she get so good?" If she keeps a guest book on her nightstand, get a clue.

If you wake up at her place one morning and see the Dallas Cowboys making breakfast, call a cab.

If she's on the Frequent Flyer plan at the Motel 6, you're not the first.

If she's starring on Spectravision in "Phallus in Wonderland," consult your physician.

A DISTURBING TREND

Girls have virtually caught up with boys in math and science performance, but they are now smoking, drinking, and using drugs as often as boys their age. That's equality for you. Although girls are not nearly as violent as boys, they are increasingly more likely to find their way into trouble with the law.

FACTS

- Sixty percent of the men cheat in America. The rest cheat in Europe. I know this because I heard it on "Jeopardy."

- Forty percent of American men experience sexual difficulties when they're exhausted, when they've had too much to drink, when they're having problems at work. How many have used these excuses?

- Twenty percent of American adults have had group sex. I don't mean to be an orgy pooper, but where I grew up, group sex was when you had a partner. Oral sex was when you talked about it.

We have books to tell us if we're good in bed. I think it's nice if they just show up and promise not to laugh. You're not good in bed if the phrase constructive criticism comes up.

BE A DAD THEY CAN TALK TO

On the plus side, we can thank Dr. Ruth, Dr. Phil, and their colleagues for opening the doors to candid conversation about sexual issues. In the seventies no one talked about condoms because birth control pills seemed to cover it, so to speak. The last time condoms were popular was in the sixties when I was growing up with no idea what they were for. I was a late bloomer who couldn't figure out what to do with his gum on his first kiss. At the age of 15 I had a friend who worked in a drugstore and used to steal boxes of rubbers and distribute them to his buddies every Friday night.

"How many do you want?" One guy would say, "I'll take two." Another guy would take three, another guy five. We called him the Wad. When it came to my turn, I didn't want to admit my naïveté and quickly said, "I'll take a dozen." That made such a huge impression that by the next Friday I said, "20." Then "30." My friends were suspicious, but by the end of the summer I had four million contraceptives. The other guys all had girlfriends and big smiles, and I had pimples and four million lover covers. (Other favorite pet names included pecker checkers and weenie warmers . . . I still had no clue!) These things were stuffed not just in my dresser drawers but in my shoes, my lunch pail, and under the rug. Some kids collected baseball cards; I collected condoms. Firestone didn't have that much rubber. I could have made my own blimp and a Trojan horse out of real Trojans. I remember coming

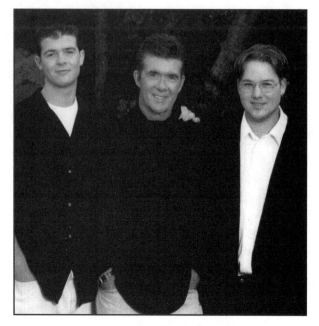

With Robin and Brennan

home one afternoon and walking into my room when the door slammed behind me. I heard the voice of God, my father, who art in cardiac arrest, standing there all red-faced and menacing with that look that fathers get when you've either brought home a lousy report card or he's found four million condoms in your drawer. I'd seen him happier. He pulled out a handful and said, "What are these?" As a doctor, I thought he should have known. When he asked, "What are they for?" I told him. Fortunately, I was way off. Something about water bombs. These turned out to be rhetorical questions since he knew very well what they were for and told me to get rid of the entire stash and, if he ever caught me with another one, I'd be sorry. I was already sorry because I sensed that would be the last conversation we would have on the subject of sex. After Dad's tirade, if I had questions about it, he wasn't the guy I would ask, and that was a loss for both of us.

There are many issues for which you'll need answers and policies as your child grows up. How tough will you be about homework? What approach will you use in discipline? Do you believe in corporal punishment? Deprivation? Authoritarian tough love or cosmic understanding? But none will affect them more than your teachings about the birds and the bees. Incidentally, if you actually refer to it as "the birds and the bees," they will never listen to you again. How many of us really knows how birds or bees do it, and who really cares? If I start doing it like a bird or a bee, stop me and turn me on to another hobby.

When we yuppies were growing up, morals were simple: put two dollars in the collection plate and stay away from barnyard animals. Girls got in trouble for premarital softball. I say kids should stay away from sex until they're old enough to appreciate the guilt and shame that go along with it. If your sons want to experience sex, let them slide down the banister like we did. Ok, enough silly. If you really want to know what's going on with them—and you will—they must feel confident discussing intimate matters with you. Parents must be the reliable consultants from day one . . . it's too important a job to be left to anyone else.

P.S.—OH, YEAH, THE KID

Your fetus now weighs a pound and a half, and, having made it past 26 weeks, the baby would probably be able to survive in a neonatal intensive care unit.

STRETCH MARK UPDATE

Around the beginning of the third trimester, a cousin to the stretch mark may appear as a dark line running down from the navel to the pubic bone. This will come as a surprise since it's probably been a while since you've been near the pubic bone. The *linea nigra* phenomenon is caused by hormonal changes and should disappear six months to a year after the baby is born. Otherwise, plan to add more lines and play hangman.

MORE FACTS

- **Hiplock: Mom's cartilage is stiffening, and you're about to see your graceful, elegant, exotic dancer-wife at her clumsiest. Gina looked like she had picked up some moves from the early Jerry Lewis movies. One night in her seventh month while having a last-chance dinner by candlelight in our bedroom, she set her robe on fire and began racing hysterically through the room** and around the bathroom—a flaming ball of pregnant madness bouncing off the walls, screaming, and looking for a place to put herself out. I tried to help, but she was unrestrainable. By the time I tossed her in the shower, her hair was singed. It's easy to laugh now . . . come to think of it, it was pretty easy to laugh then. She'll kill me for this anecdote, so pretend you heard it from the housekeeper.

FACTS

- Eighty-six percent of American women think there is too much emphasis on sex today. Only 66 percent of American men agree.

- A survey of 10,000 adults by the University of Chicago studied who gets the most sex. If you're a couch potato who listens to jazz, owns a gun, votes liberal, smokes, drinks, and makes less than $30,000 a year, congratulations!

- Only one mother in seven actually gets around to telling her kids about sex.

- Teenagers learn most about sex from friends, followed by TV, parents, and sex ed.

- The average age at first intercourse is 17 for girls and 16 for boys.

- What women first notice about men:
    Clothing—33 percent
    Face—31 percent
    Body—20 percent
    Hair—17 percent
    Height—10 percent

- Wanna fall out of love? Your body has 10 gallons of water sloshing around inside, along with a sea of organisms, cells, and bacteria. Your have enough fat for 6 cakes of soap, phosphorus for 212 matches, carbon for 28 pounds of coal, and iron for a 1-inch nail. Sounds like a blind date with Lake Erie.

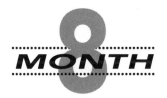

MONTH 8

FOOTSTEPS

Now in the eighth month, your angel-in-waiting has all the hair with which he or she will be born and can distinguish different shades of light. I was curious at learning the latter, having presumed that lighting conditions in the womb would be fairly consistent . . . dark! For more info, consult your doctor or electrician.

Meanwhile, if your doctor shines that fetoscope light inside the uterus, your baby's eyes are now sensitive enough that its hands will try to shield them.

Your fetus is now practicing breathing by inhaling amniotic fluid. I don't remember what amniotic fluid tastes like, but presumably it's the kind of thing you'd want to try only as a fetus and not make your beverage of choice at the fraternity.

Mom will be tested for Group B streptococcus bacteria this month and if she tests positive will likely be treated with penicillin and given an antibiotic during childbirth to protect the baby from infection. The bacteria lurks harmlessly in about 30 percent of women's bodies, but approximately 8,000 American newborns are infected at birth every year, 800 die, and up to half suffer long-term damage from seizures.

With one month to go, Mom will want to simply sit or lie in whatever comfortable position she can find—a tough job because there isn't one. You'll think she's solar-powered because the only time she moves is when the sun is in her face.

The baby weighs about four pounds and is moving into its birth position. Mom's cartilage is loosening to allow her pelvic bones more flexibility in delivery.

In one of those miracles that God planted in our physiognomy, he included some helpful hormones for the hips—technically known as the "helpful hip hormones"—that cause muscles around the hips to relax, creating more room for the baby to exit. The hip joints may have a loosey-goosey feel, and when you combine this with late-natal weight gain and backache—footsteps month is also backache month—that accounts for her new walk, the unmistakable pregnant waddle. The male equivalent of the pregnant waddle is a 325-pound defensive tackle trying to drag his butt back to the line of scrimmage late in the game on a hot day in Miami without passing out.

At 36 weeks the baby is likely to drop or engage in the pelvis, creating more space for Mom's lungs and stomach and some relief from the shortness of breath and heartburn. The bad news is that her bladder capacity is now smaller than ever, and if you can't imagine her peeing more often, know that the toilet will barely flush before she needs it again.

There may be some increased vaginal discharge, soiling your bed sheets and your loved one's underwear. Women have a fine instinct for personal hygiene and propriety that makes them uncomfortable about sharing their little messes with anyone else. Men have no such embarrassment over soiled underwear, which no doubt came as a shock to your wife when you first started living together. It would serve you right if she left her undergarment in a place where you'd see it and go "ooh, yuck." In a tribute to her unfailing dignity, however, she will more likely clean up after herself and save you the experience.

"I'M BORED"

Encourage her to continue her daily routine, but nothing too strenuous and certainly no heavy lifting. I'm sure it's been a while since she changed a tire or held those shingles while you roofed, but if you've let it go this long, it can wait.

"ANYTHING BUT THOSE STUPID MAGIC TRICKS"

You can pitch in by helping arrange her schedule and providing enough entertainment to keep her occupied while her mother shingles the roof. This is a fine time to knit or needlepoint if she is so inclined. Does she like crossword puzzles? Many women take that spiritual inspiration and turn it into creative literature by writing poetry or even children's stories. Surround her with her favorite videos. Some titles that appeal to an expectant mother are *Out of Africa, Dr. Zhivago, Nine Months*, and *She's Having a Baby*. Less appropriate titles would include *Mommie Dearest, The Hand That Rocks the Cradle*, and *Sophie's Choice*.

PONDERABLES: "CAN I STUMP YOU JUST ONCE?"

To entertain and distract the truly creative pregnant thinker, try these on for size.

- **Why do they bother putting an expiration date on sour cream?**

- **When shipping Styrofoam, what do you pack it in?**

- **What do you send a surrogate mother on Mother's Day? Artificial flowers?**

- **In which direction does a Jewish dyslexic read?**

- **Do you realize there is no other word for thesaurus?**

- **When a ventriloquist performs oral sex, does he move his lips?**

- **Why did kamikaze pilots bother wearing helmets?**

- **If they have a vote to legalize marijuana, would it be called a reeferendum?**

Her new spiritual awareness may inspire her to challenge you with, "What kind of a world are we leaving our children?" You have no quick answer fro this one, except to say that we all miss Frank Sinatra and baseball games are too long.

Don't be surprised at your own depth when you find yourself thinking weightier thoughts than ever before. You will soon have an important reason to live a long and healthy life, a purpose beyond saving up to buy that boat.

A BIG PROJECT

Both of you will muse about family trees, ancestry, heritage, ethnicity, and legacy as you hit the stretch run. (Oops! The "s" word again.) The baby industry will be only too happy to sell you Baby's First Scrapbook, Baby's First Photo Album, Baby's First Guest Book; they'll bronze his first shoe and petrify his first poop. Stock up now on the keepsake holders; you'll want to document the first weeks of life. I collected a stack of magazines and newspapers that appeared the same week Carter did. You get only one chance at those souvenirs, and if family sentiment is important, you'll be glad you were prepared.

Start putting together the family album you've been working on for three years because every picture you take from now on will be of your child. One day it will be great fun to have all the great grandparents and weird uncles lined up in photo form to greet your baby from those hallowed pages. You can't wait to teach him the connection between his future and his past, and if you climb your family tree, I know you'll find some nuts that will entertain your newcomer and give him a sense of belonging to the lineage he's joining.

I first learned the importance of family from my parents, who, coincidentally, were in my family.

My brother, Todd, and his wife, Marybeth, were expecting around the same time as Gina and me, a fortuitous coincidence guaranteeing that our babies would have a same-age cousin to play with. Let's be honest, compete with! The cousin friendship/rivalry will actually be a thinly disguised competition between brothers, Todd and me, so let the games begin! The handsome and fabulous Evan Jack Brian Thicke was born first. Damn, they beat us on that one! When Evan was eight pounds eight ounces, I knew our kid would have to come in at eight pounds nine ounces, and I began feeding Gina accordingly. Meanwhile, her ultrasound picture had to be clearer, her back spasms more painful, her feet more swollen, and so on. We could only hope that the cousins would be bright enough to ignore the primitive relationship we were setting up with this irksome internecine one-upsmanship.

BY THE WAY . . .

Our Carter William was born at seven pounds one ounce, disappointingly short of cousin Evan's bulk. Six of those pounds, however, were penis, accompanied by a world-class scrotum so oversized that, in fact, it had to be delivered separately two days later. Take that, little brother!

"WHY, WHEN I WAS YOUR AGE . . ."

I suggest writing about your hometown memories for your baby's keepsake book.

Me? I'm glad you asked. I was born in Kirkland Lake, a small, remote town in the far north of Ontario, Canada. That cold mass that's always coming down to the eastern states begins in Kirkland Lake. It's not the end of the world, but you can see it from there. You arrive by canoe, and a beaver takes your bags. The best-looking girl in town was an inflatable. Kirkland Lake was a mining town, once reputed to have the deepest shaft in North America. (Could be a Viagra joke.) I worked summers in a uranium mine, which is why I have five testicles today.

I did a few hometown jokes on *The Tonight Show*, and the townspeople got so mad at me (all six of them), someone threatened to tar and feather my grandmother. She said the feather part sounded interesting.

Okay, I'm sorry if I've painted a bleak picture of my hometown. But I was only trying to stimulate tourism, and it worked—a family flocked there just last year. My name was in the running for the naming of a new park in town . . . until the "inflatable girl" joke. As luck would have it, there's now a new celebrity from the area after whom they can name things. Kirkland Lake is now "The Home of Shania Twain and Alan Who?" She's in; I'm out. They're having a parade for her and a pig barbecue for me.

THE TRUTH

My grandparents contributed a great deal to the fine community of Kirkland Lake and to its unique character by the places they worked, the buildings they built, the children they raised, and the changes they made. Our grandparents paved the way for the good life we enjoy, and we owe them repayment in kind for a debt we can never repay in full. My grandparents were saints, and all they ever had they gave to us. Their names were Isadora and Willis Greer, but we always called them Is and Will. I've donated the annual Willis Greer Scholarship Award at the Kirkland Lake High School to the senior student who does the most to help senior citizens.

Will was proud of that.

The following observations about grandmothers came from the mouths of babes to cyberspace and, once again, are either public domain or someone out there may sue for plagiarism. Take your best shot.

- **Grandmothers are ladies who have no children of their own so they like other people's boys and girls to play with.**

- **Usually, they are fat and wear glasses and funny underwear. They can take their teeth and gums off.**

- **When they take us for walks, they go slow past things like pretty leaves and caterpillars, and they never tell us to hurry up.**

- **When they read to us, they don't skip words and they don't mind if it's the same old story.**

- **Grandmas are the only grown-ups who have time.**

- **Remember . . . try to teach your kids something every day. It will usually be the same thing you tried to teach them yesterday.**

- **You're only young once, but you can be immature forever.**

- **When the chips are down, you can count your real friends on one hand. You can express your feelings for the others on one finger.**

- **Things happen for a reason. That reason is to piss you off.**

One lesson I would recommend passing on to your kids: *Follow your dream, but don't be a dreamer.* In other words, pursue your goals, but be willing to adjust and compromise if, after a reasonable time, reality tells you, "Hey pal . . . at 4'10", you'll be a better jockey than a point guard!" Push the envelope but then accept your limitations. For those with show biz fantasies— and many of your children will have them—there are plenty of ways to be fulfilled other than being a movie star. Behind the cameras there is production, public relations, commercial sales, teaching, and amateur theater, all of which can get you a piece of the dream. I'm certain this philosophy applies to most pursuits.

EXCEPTION TO THE RULE

Do not follow your dream if it involves bagpipes. I took pipe lessons as a teen and became a lonely geek overnight. But I digress.

FACTS

- The stress hormone, cortisol, rises dramatically in late pregnancy.

- There are 30 times as many people buried in the earth as are now living on it.

- In 1901, a man's life expectancy was 48 years; a woman's, 51.

- By 2005, there will be more than 100,000 Americans aged 100 or older.

- The average woman talks much more about other people than about anything else. Men tend to talk most about work.

- Best places to live:
    - For work and family: Seattle
    - For business: Utah
    - For women: San Francisco
    - For retirement: Las Vegas

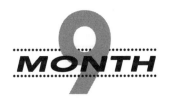

MONTH 9

TOUCHDOWN!

A USC study shows that Mom's intellectual functioning is diminished in the weeks before delivery because women's brains temporarily shrink. Now they tell us! Obstetrical nurses call it pregnancy brain, and the resulting fuzzy-headedness can make it difficult to remember the day of the week or where you left your keys.

Performance during pregnancy was 20 percent lower on the skills tested than performance after childbirth. More than 70 percent of the women had difficulty learning new information during their ninth month.

MVP

Regardless of how politically correct we are on the subject of equality of the sexes, the one undeniable fact of life that separates us is that women are still having the babies.

No matter how even we are in the boardroom or at the pool table, only one of us will be pushing a pumpkin out of her stomach. Only one of us has been bombarded by the hormones from hell for eight months, and we husbands should take a moment to savor the heroism of our mate. The strength and courage and love and caring that she has put into this project are the stuff of greatness. Those of us born before the women's movement remember the bias against women who only had children, only raised a family, only managed a household—the only implying that these pursuits were somehow less important than an out-of-home job with a paycheck.

For all the advances our world has made economically and technologically, we still see increases in crime, domestic violence, child abuse, and divorce. Do we need more mothering? The pendulum is swinging back to the middle between the two extremes of career women and nonincome mothers, recognizing that the important decision for moms on whether to work or not to work—or when to work or how much—is a personal choice. The key is to do what's right for your goals, your marriage, and your family.

The frustrating thing about motherhood is when do you know if you've done a good job? When is it over? When have you been enough? Done enough? Surely you are not a successful mother simply because you give birth to a healthy baby. Will you be successful if your daughter has gone off to her first day of school equipped with nice manners and the names of all the states? When she graduates from high school without making an attempt on your life or getting pregnant herself, is your mother job complete? When she's elected president of the United States? The answer is an unequivocal no. Hopefully never. Parenting is a life-long activity, responsibility, opportunity, and blessing.

With the impending birth of my third son, I had many friends marvel, "Wow, you're starting all over again!" As true as that may be, the other reality is that I've never stopped. The older our children get, the higher go the stakes. The big decision for the new baby is whether to feed him peas or carrots tonight, whether to dress him in the blue outfit or the green one tomor-row. Now every decision the older ones make is momentous: What to drive, whom to date, where to live, where to work, when to "just say no" to the temp-tations confronting them in the world outside my doors.

Who could argue that motherhood isn't the most important job in the world and one of the toughest? A mother will be doing her job at 3:00 in the morning for many more nights than a doctor will. A mother will have to balance a budget with the skill of a corporate CEO. The mother of a 9-year-old boy may see more actual combat than a five-star general. The mother of a 15-year-old girl will have to keep her eye on more men than a yard guard at Attica. Our hats go off to the women who combine motherhood with a career outside the home, but if it ever comes to an either/or choice, don't let anybody tell you that punching a clock or winning a promotion is more significant than tending to your son or daughter.

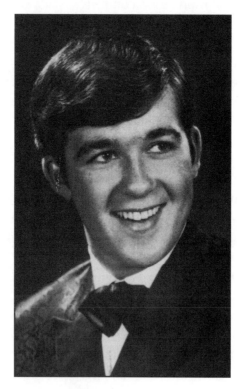

Geeks have babies, too!

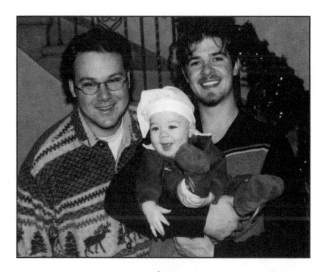

My three sons:
Brennan Todd, Carter William, and Robin Alan

R-E-S-P-E-C-T

- 86 percent of moms think they don't get enough respect and that moms who stay at home get even less and working moms look down on them. Even so, 77 percent of mothers who work full-time would rather stay home if they could.

- 70 percent of mothers say that being a mom is much more demanding than they expected, 92 percent say it is also much more rewarding.

FROM A MOM ON THE INTERNET

Renewing my driver's license, I was self-conscious about listing "mother" as an occupation.

"Do you have a job?" the clerk inquired.

"I'm a . . . research associate in the field of child development and human relations."

"Might I ask just what you do in your field?"

"I have a continuing program of research (what mother doesn't?) in the laboratory and in the field. I'm working for my masters (the whole darned family) and already have four credits (all daughters). Of course, the job is one of the most demanding in the humanities (any mother care to disagree?), and I often work 14 hours a day (24 is more like it). But the job is more challenging than most run-of-the-mill careers, and the rewards are in satisfaction rather than just money."

As I drove into our driveway, impressed by my glamorous new career, I was greeted by my lab assistants—ages 13, 7, and 3. Upstairs, I could hear our new experimental model (six months) in the child-development program, testing out a new vocal pattern. I felt triumphant. I had scored a point on bureaucracy and was now in the official records as someone more distinguished and indispensable to mankind than "just another mother . . ."

HERE WE GO!

Ladies . . . four million women give birth in the United States every year. You are about to be one of them.

This is it. This is what it's all about. You're in the bigs, at the dance, the shot clock running down, it's the two-minute drill, bottom of the ninth, sudden-death overtime, and several other sports clichés apropos of this moment.

If *How Men Have Babies* is the only pregnancy book you've read to this point, I am flattered and you are screwed. The baby could arrive any day now, any minute. You might not even get to finish this month. Are you truly ready to hear "Let's go"?

Your wife's uterus has expanded to a thousand times its original size. Men cannot relate to any such occurrence in their own genitalia, Viagra jokes notwithstanding.

The fetus is doing crazy things, like swallowing the downy lanugo and waxy vernix that lodge in the baby's bowels and become the child's first bowel movement (meconium).

The vaginal tract will secrete fluids similar to urine, yeast infection, or bag of waters. This is a good thing to know and a horrible thing to be surprised by. These are fluids used by and no longer useful to the fetus.

Frankly, the birth business could use a little help in the public relations department. Any theatrical production that described its final act in terms like mucous plug and bloody show would be fighting an uphill battle. This describes *Macbeth*, not *A Funny Thing Happened on the Way to the Maternity Ward*. Why couldn't *mucous plug* be the *dam of dampness*? Why not *crimson caper* for *bloody show*?

You may hear "let's go" before it's really time since it is not uncommon for mothers to have weeks of false labor, although why anyone would want to fake such a thing ranks right up there with becoming a mother at 61. If you were taking notes in Month 5, you would know that only 1 in 20 hit the predicted due date on the nose. If you are more than two weeks late, your OB/GYN will consider you overdue, chicken, or stubborn.

Expect to see the Braxton-Hicks phenomenon: prelabor contractions that feel like indigestion or menstrual cramps, sometimes accompanied by diarrhea.

Women: if you think you are experiencing true labor, call your doctor and report when your contractions started, how long they're lasting, how far you are from the hospital, and whether or not your husband is still conscious.

The doctor will want to know if the bag of waters has broken, but keep in mind that this rupturing of the amniotic membrane signals the beginning of true labor only about 15 percent of the time.

Although you know that Fright Night is near, the only way to be certain about real labor is to have your cervix checked. I'm sure women would agree it would be a brilliant invention if medical science could come up with an implant lodged in the uterus that would call your phone number when true labor begins. This would be called an answering cervix. That was a long way to go for that joke, so thanks for bearing with me.

ACCORDING TO VANNA

I spent the last few days of pregnancy floating in the pool. When you are a week late, you feel like a whale, so why not spend it like one! I had been having minor labor pains for two weeks. . . . I was so ready! (All women should add at least one week to their due date so when the baby is late they won't feel let down like I was.) I've heard how miserable you are the last two weeks. You feel fat, full, uncomfortable, a little depressed and emotional. But the good news is, the end is near, and that's what keeps you going. Then when you meet your new bundle of joy, you will see it was definitely worth the wait!

VANNA WHITE, MOTHER OF GIOVANNA

KATHIE LEE—ARMED AND DANGEROUS

During the last two weeks of my pregnancy with Cassidy, I was in the miserable throes of false labor and experiencing all the joy of delivery with no delivery! I have never been more anxious and more frustrated, more anguished or more evil than during this period. It was the middle of July, and I felt as though I would boil over and explode.

At one point while I was groaning in my bed, Frank had the audacity, no the courage, to say to me, "Oh, come on, Golda, you're just faking it." I got out of bed, got in the car, drove into town, and screeched around the underground parking lot of the movie theater for two hours. It was the only thing that saved me from a life behind bars for murdering my husband. Nevertheless, I have a fantasy that at my sentencing I'd look into the benevolent and understanding face of a female judge—a woman! Better yet, a mother! "Not guilty," she would pronounce with a smack from her gavel and a gleam in her eye.

KATHIE LEE GIFFORD

The most common sign of true labor is that she will lose her mucous plug. Around this point you may also lose your car keys, lose your way to the hospital, and lose the doctor's phone number. This is called losing it. Fortunately, that kind of panic is usually reserved for movie comedies and, in fact, it is not necessary to rush to the hospital, even at the first signs of labor.

Your doctor may actually encourage you to stay home for the early stages because your relaxation is important. Soft lighting, soft music, and a husbandly massage might help both of you. It is not recommended that she eat, but drinking clear fluids is fine.

Walking around is advised because false contractions will usually dissipate whereas contractions that intensify will be an indication that this is the real thing. Either way, being upright will help, and your doctor might even have you walk around at the hospital, waiting for more dilation.

In birth class you learned that one of your important roles is to time the contractions. They will start at 15, 20, even 30 minutes apart, and when looking for the next sign, remember the phrase "longer and stronger." This may be one of the ways you described yourself to your wife when you were dating, but now longer and stronger is how you count contractions. When they come five minutes apart, lasting a minute, and making it difficult for her to walk and talk while she's having one, it's time to put your bags in the car and pretend you're calm and in charge.

How much dilation before we get in the car? How much dilation before the epidural? Have you done your homework?

WHAT TO PACK FOR THE HOSPITAL

1. **Warm socks**

2. **Hair barrettes**

3. **Lip balm**

4. **Breath spray**

5. **Magazines**

6. **Music**

7. **Something to play it on (CD or cassette player; no bagpipes)**

8. Gas for the car

9. Snacks for the coach—so he's not at the vending machine when the kid hits the fan

10. And, oh yes . . . be sure to bring the wife

FROM JERRY HALL

"Mick [Jagger] arrived at the hospital bearing diamond earrings and caviar. The wives and nurses were very excited to find him there with a pot of caviar, asking if they had some lemon slices and toast."

ENTERTAINMENT WEEKLY

This was apparently one of the more amusing memories Jerry had of their marriage.

Until now, your co-procreator has been in the latent phase of labor, resting up for the active phase, when cervical dilation is around four centimeters. Dilation will increase at one to two centimeters per hour, and when contractions happen every three minutes, you should be seeing your baby in six to ten hours.

DRUGS

My hero, Dave Barry, who writes funnier than anyone in the English language, made these observations
in *Playboy* magazine (May 1990):

> There are two systems for childbirth. There's the
> old system, under which I was born, where the man did
> not have to watch. That was a good system. The man's
> function was to sit in the waiting room and read old
> copies of *Field & Stream* and smoke a lot of Camels. As
> for the woman, she did have to be in the delivery
> room—but she was given extensive narcotics and did-
> n't wake up until the child was entering the third grade.
>
> The only people who actually had to watch the baby
> come out were trained medical personnel wearing masks
> and getting paid for it. But later, in the mid-seventies,
> without any legislation being passed that I know of, the
> man was suddenly required to go and watch the baby
> being born! Not only that but there were even classes
> where we sat around in a room with people we didn't
> know and discussed things like the uterus. (There was a
> time in my life when I would have killed for reliable infor-
> mation about the uterus. But having discussed it in detail,
> and having seen actual full-color pictures of it, while I
> respect it a great deal as an organ, it's lost a lot of its
> sparkle for me.)
>
> Anyway, in these classes, they kept talking about
> "contractions." They never used the word pain. So
> when the great day came and the baby was actually
> coming out, Beth was making noises like a whale, and
> she tried the breathing exercises and they were really

effective for, oh, I'd say 15, possibly even 20 seconds. Then she switched to the more traditional method, which is screaming for drugs.

Thanks, Dave.

DRUG DATA

- **Under the new laws in California, marijuana is legal for emergency medical purposes. The breaking of the bag of waters may qualify as such a moment for expectant fathers.**

- **Twenty-five percent of American women who give birth receive an epidural to help them cope with their pain.**

There are pluses and minuses to taking medication. Since walking can help speed labor, you don't want her legs too numb to stand up. On the other hand, medication does decrease pain. Medication could reduce the muscle sensation required to push the baby out, which might slow things down to the point that forceps or even a cesarean is necessary. On the other hand, medication decreases pain. Narcotics can interfere with the baby's breathing if they're administered too late in labor. On the plus side, medication decreases pain. Some experts are convinced that medication during labor can interfere with the baby's first nursing instincts. Still, medication decreases pain. You could have a hungover feeling the next day. Nevertheless . . . you get the picture.

Know the difference between narcotics and anesthetics. Anesthetics are to ease pain. Narcotics can get you 18 months.

A narcotic shot—to sedate nervousness—takes about 40 minutes to kick in fully. A 40-minute window could seem like an eternity, so anticipate and time yourself accordingly.

Anesthesiologists now typically mix small doses of narcotics with a diluted anesthetic solution. These narcotic epidurals seem to be the best of both worlds for the mother because they preserve motor function in the lower extremities. Calm and numb are two welcome feelings for the delivery room.

The combo epidural also wears off faster—after about two hours—with the goal being that her sensations are all there when it comes time to push and when push comes to shove, etc.

Doctors at the University of Texas Southwestern Medical Center found that women who received epidurals averaged nearly 8 hours in labor. Women who chose intravenous Demerol, which offers less relief from pain, averaged only 6½ hours. Labor medications rarely delayed interaction with the newborn.

If you have an epidural, try to nurse as soon as possible to restore your baby's alertness and early sucking instinct.

The journal *Pediatrics* reports that women who have epidurals experience a higher rate of fever during labor and delivery. Fever in the mother is a concern because it can indicate an infection in the baby, meaning tests for the baby, which may mean antibiotics for the baby, who then stays behind in the hospital after Mom is released, all of which will be very upsetting to new parents. Epidural-related fever, however, may simply be telling us that the mother's numbness has thrown off her temperature regulator.

Since the medical community has reached no unanimous consensus on epidural blocks and their relationship to newborn infection or C-sections, you will be required to make your own informed decision. Question your doctor thoroughly until you feel comfortable in the choice you make about anesthesia.

DO YOU KNOW A RELIABLE DEALER?

I mentioned that Gina was no martyr and easily decided that she would prefer to be numbed to the pain. What I mean is, she chose to have drugs. What I'm saying is, we should have had the baby in Colombia.

Let me go out on a limb and offer my personal choice. The percentages in the problem areas are low, the odds are on your side, and your wife should not be discouraged from relieving her pain by the possibility of complications that, to revive the sports parlance, are a long shot. If she has had a healthy pregnancy and all systems are go as you approach term, my money is on the drugs. Just try to delay the epidural until the cervix has dilated to five centimeters. The alternative could be her holding a grudge for the rest of your lives because you made her go through hell without a fire hose.

Keep in mind that, as in the schoolyard, these drugs are not free. On the contrary, when you get your hospital bill, you may think you opened escrow on a beach house. In the line item called painkiller, whatever drug they were giving you has a street value equal to the gross national product of Cameroon.

SHOW ME THE BABY!

I was trying to coach Sarah with her breathing . . . leaned in close and blew. She said, "Back off; your breath stinks." When she pleaded for the epidural, I reminded her, "Sweetheart, it's just like that pain I had when my tooth was pulled." She said, "Oh, yeah? Now imagine that tooth was in your ass!"

CUBA GOODING JR., FATHER OF SPENCER AND MASON

This is the moment of truth for you, big fella, time to swing into action with Lamaze, Bradley, or whatever method you've been practicing. The breathing, massaging, and reassuring conversation or total silence you agreed on should take place now.

Let me digress for the last time to point out that in college I actually studied premed . . . for about an hour.

For me medical school was a senseless waste of human lunch—in a word, disgusting. I was a fainter . . . sick people made me sick.

In my second year, after fainting for the third time, I decided to tell my father, the doctor, that I had to quit. Then he fainted.

The worst fainting I ever did was when my first son was born. Childbirth proved to be a good test of my pain threshold (i.e., my tolerance for someone else's discomfort). My first ex-wife and I had been studying natural childbirth, which, if truth be told, is the ultimate misnomer. There is nothing natural about the noises women make in childbirth. "ha-ee-oh-wa-chee-oh" sounded like Jackie Chan was the father of my child.

Undaunted, I was prepared to stand in the corner with the smock and a first baseman's mitt to catch the baby. "Come on, baby, fire that baby in there, baby." The first clue is, you're a bad dad if you miss and the baby hits the wall.

When the big natural childbirth moment came, I did what came naturally: I fainted! She went into labor, and I went into a coma. This came as no surprise to my wife. I had also fainted during conception.

I share this embarrassment to make the point that in the seventies, natural childbirth was so emphatically the rage that any divergence fell somewhere between *heretical* and *dangerous*. Some doctors and birth coaches used scare tactics to dissuade from any other form of delivery, including inducement of labor, the breaking of the bag of waters, anesthesia, or, worst of all, cesarean section. The threat was that the baby would experience oxygen deprivation, birth trauma, or brain damage; be unemployable; leave his room messy; wear polyester; watch Richard Gere movies; and suffer a host of other unimaginables. So conditioned was I against these alternatives that when 22 hours of labor passed and the doctor finally announced that we might need all of the above, I hit the floor like a North Hollywood bank teller.

When I came to, I heard my mother making excuses to the nurses in the hall that I'd had a long day, hadn't eaten, had low blood sugar, etc. Meanwhile, birth mother was making so much noise I could hardly pass out! A classic case of the Husband Seeking Attention Syndrome? Not on purpose, honest. It's just that the birthing community had scared me into thinking that "natural" was the only way to go. I hope our time together on these pages has assured you otherwise.

THE BON JOVI METHOD

After years of playing lead guitar in one of the world's great rock bands, Richie Sambora thought he had seen it all. But nothing, including birth class, could have prepared him for cesarean.

I've seen rockers bite the heads off chickens, but that's kid's stuff compared to the sci-fi movie they call cesarean birth. When the doctor cauterized the veins and smoke started billowing from Heather's stomach, I knew this would be an awesome show. I got queasy when I saw parts of my wife I had never seen before resting on her lap. But I had confidence that this was all routine for the doctors when I heard them discussing the USC football game. The whole thing was surreal. And, no, you won't find any home movies of the birth on the Internet.

RICHIE SAMBORA, FATHER OF AVA

HAIL, CAESAR!

- **In the '80s C-sections comprised a quarter of all deliveries**

- **C-sections may help prevent the transmission of HIV infection and genital herpes, but critics worried about infections and hemorrhaging**

- **The latest figures on VBAC (Vaginal Birth After Cesarean) indicate that 70 percent of women who tried this have successful births without resorting to surgery**

- **The maternal mortality rate is 2 to 4 times greater in a cesarean than in a vaginal birth**

- **The Caesar Salad was actually invented in Mexico**

At eight or nine centimeters of dilation, you will be entering the transition stage of labor, where the baby is descending farther down the birth canal and contractions can last up to a minute and a half. At this point the doctor will perform a vaginal exam and feel the baby's head. Until now, the mother's focus has been on withstanding the pain, but she now has to get into the game and perform. It's time to start pushing, using her own musculature to exit the baby. The pushing period can be short, if you're lucky, and last two or three hours if you're typical.

In this second and final stage of labor, the baby is under more stress, so fetal monitoring is crucial. I will never forget the sight of the top of Carter William's wet and hairy little head poking out as my first view of him. He was a furry little guy with a generous scalpful, meaning later in life he should have the option of a blow-dried, feathered look as opposed to that matted-down yarmulke he started with. This first breathtaking glimpse will be one of the truly uncontrollable emotional moments of your life. This is where you as a father finally have a leg up on your beloved—while she has two legs up on the world—because unless you play tricks with mirrors at the foot of the bed, you are going to see this marvel before your wife does. It seems unfair after she did all the work, but that is the first of many great privileges in being a father.

It is at this point you are short of breath, your sinuses fill up, your stomach is in your throat, your heart is racing, and it will be impossible not to shed a tear. If you don't cry now, you're not human. Whatever speech you had planned for this moment will go out the window. I remember saying simply, "He's coming . . . he's coming . . . he's here!" You are witnessing the most awesome display of God's special effects imaginable.

I was sane enough to grab the video camera and start documenting Carter's life while the doctor did his thing. As referenced in an earlier month, this was great progress for me, having fainted with one son, having survived the second, and having spent 20 years learning how to operate a camcorder. I got close-ups, wide angles, zooms, and pans and used most of the techniques that make you dizzy when you watch MTV. Very contemporary. Very artistic.

It can be shocking to see the doctor pull your baby's head out and twist it 180 degrees like a plastic doll. I hope you've seen photographs of this procedure and the way a baby looks in the first 15 seconds of life so that you won't be horrified by the blue-gray, drenched, lifeless appearance. He looks like a prop from the *Alien* movies, and you're anxious to hear the doctor tell you everything is fine because there is no obvious sign of life with the eyes closed and no breathing or crying.

"HOWIE MANDEL" SHOW, AUGUST 27, 1998

ALAN:

*If you have another little anecdote anywhere
near as disgusting as that feather in the butt
thing, I want to use it . . .*

HOWIE:

*I can think of one. My wife got mad at me in the
birthing room because her legs were in stirrups
and her knees were up and my first daughter,
Jackie, was making her way out . . . and the
head came out. And I started laughing . . .
because just the image of just a head hanging
out of the bottom of my wife . . . it looked like
just a really bad puppet show. I told my wife
that and then she said, "Get out."*

ALAN:

Just sign this release form . . .

The twisting of the head is done to clear the air passages, and the doctor will quickly remove mucus from the mouth and nostrils so by the time the rest of the body shoots out, he or she will take that first breath and begin crying and the world will be a brighter place than you've ever seen!

You may have discussed the cutting of the umbilical cord and decided you would like to participate in that ceremony. The doctor and nurse will clean up your baby first, and within minutes you will get to do the honors. It's an easy matter, and you can even continue running your video with one hand while cutting with the other. (As thrilled as your wife is with sharing this moment, she may not want any further responsibility, like holding the camera. Don't push your luck; it's going great so far!)

There is yet another stage, devoted to the expulsion of the placenta.

Fact: The placenta is delivered shortly after the baby and looks like a large pancake made of tissue and blood vessels. This will change your feelings about pancakes forever.

Fact: They use placenta in the manufacture of shampoos. You can sign donation papers if you wish. Odds are that's not the first thing you women think about when you've delivered a baby. "Is it a boy or a girl? And don't forget to save my placenta for Paul Mitchell."

This is the cleanup operation, and it's important for Dad to follow through and help out and not be off handing out phallic cigars while the missus is stuck with the mess. The placenta may be expelled naturally with a little assistance from the obstetrician, who will regard this phase as critical, lest the placenta become trapped inside the uterus or the mother lose too much blood. After the extraction of the placenta, most hospitals will give the mother pitocin to make the uterus contract.

Remember months ago when she showed restraint in exposing you to her new bodily functions? This was because she knew full well that at the moment of delivery, she expects to gross you out with an unforgettable display of insides being turned out, and gore to the max that could take six months from which to recover. The baby may be a year old before you can look at those body parts again with the same panting enthusiasm you felt when you first saw them. (Having you in the delivery room is her clever way of guaranteeing that you won't get too sexed up in the foreseeable future.)

The final steps will be to check that the uterus is firm, that the bleeding is minimal, and that any tears or lacerations are stitched up if needed, as in "please repair the episiotomy."

Also, do you stay with mother or child while the nurse cleans up? Fear of the "switched at birth" syndrome comes into play here. What tests and shots have you planned for the newborn? What about circumcision? (Note: This is the only aspect of childbirth about which there is absolutely nothing funny. Don't even try. I had visions of a Benihana chef trimming my kid.)

For mom, be prepared for lochia—the bloody vaginal discharge that can last for six weeks afterward, described by some as a heavy period and by others as a vampire movie.

UGLY BABIES

Once you know he's healthy, the next thing you scrutinize is his looks. It's true, looks aren't important . . . unless they're bad ones. Prepare to start stifling yourself in the bragging area, because despite all of the complaints and commotion, through all of the sarcasm and silliness, one truth will prevail: your child is the most brilliant, most coordinated, most mature, most talented, most beautiful baby ever to see the light of day on God's green earth. In many cases, this is hyperbole. (My own children happen to be the rare exception and, as luck would have it, are genuinely gifted and gorgeous.)

The tendency will be to take your child to the mall or the park and point fingers and laugh smugly at the ugly babies. This is an unkind and sorry example to set for your child but irresistible nonetheless.

"CONGRATULATIONS, IT'S A . . . ?"

You're a father! And at this moment the happiest man in the world, having the most amazing day of his life! Words fail me, and coming up with them is my job, so you probably won't do much better. Things like "Thank God!" and "Hello, precious!" come to mind and will do nicely. Your life will never be the same, and your existence will never have more meaning. You suddenly, clearly see why you were born—so you could have him . . . *or her!!* And as for Mom . . .

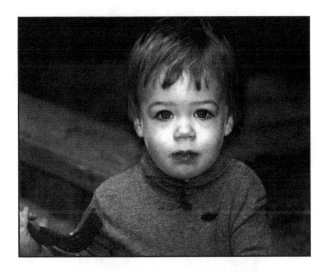

*"Write any caption you want,
but I have nothing on my mind."*

SORRY RUDYARD!

If you can keep your head when all about you
Are losing theirs in the delivery room
If you can breathe and push and sometimes shout, you
Will get what you've got coming from your womb
If you can take the pain for one more minute
And save your tears for when the job is done
You'll have the world and everything that's in it
And best, you'll have a daughter or a son!

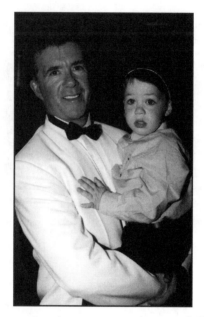

"Dad always has his maitre d job to fall back on."

GOD HELP US ALL!

I'll say good-bye now because I know you're busy with baby stuff.

May all your baby dreams come true.

May your child be blessed with health and happiness.

May you feel each other's love always.

May you bump into me one day with your child in tow and say hello. . . . I'll say "I knew him when. . . ."

All the best . . .
Love, Alan

ABOUT THE AUTHOR

ALAN THICKE is a seven-time Emmy Award-nominated actor, writer, and a Golden Globe nominee for his role as psychiatrist and father, Jason Seaver, from TV's *Growing Pains*. He has written TV specials for Bill Cosby, Flip Wilson, and Richard Pryor, among others, as well as the revolutionary comedies *"Fernwood 2-Night"* and *"America 2-Night."* Alan Made his Broadway debut in 1998 starring as lawyer Billy Flynn in *Chicago—The Musical*. His experience as an entertainer includes acting, writing, and producing, spanning television, film, concerts and theater. He has been honored as "Father of the Year" by a number of family-themed charities, and his proudest role remains father to his three sons, Brennan, Robin, and Carter.

We hope this Jodere Group book has benefited you in your quest for personal, intellectual, and spiritual growth.

Jodere Group is passionate about bringing new and exciting books, such as HOW MEN HAVE BABIES, to readers worldwide. Our company was created as a unique publishing and multi-media avenue for individuals whose mission it is to positively impact the lives of others. We recognize the strength of an original thought, a kind word and a selfless act—and the power of the individuals who possess them. We are committed to providing the support, passion, and creativity necessary for these individuals to achieve their goals and dreams.

Jodere Group is comprised of a dedicated and creative group of people who strive to provide the highest quality of books, audio programs, online services, and live events to people who pursue life-long learning. It is our personal and professional commitment to embrace our authors, speakers, and readers with helpfulness, respect, and enthusiasm.

**For more information
about our products, authors, or live events,
please call (800) 569-1002
or visit us on the Web at
www.jodere.com**

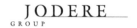

JODERE
GROUP